# *Hurry Up Nurse 2*

**DAWN BROOKES**

# *Hurry Up Nurse 2*

*London Calling*

By

**DAWN BROOKES**

DAWN BROOKES PUBLISHING

*Published by DAWN BROOKES PUBLISHING*
*www.dawnbrookespublishing.com*

Paperback Edition 2017
ISBN: 978-0-9955561-4-0

Cover Design by Janet Dado

*This one is for Jenny*

# Contents

# Preface

This book contains a collection of memories from my experiences of a training course I undertook following my initial Enrolled Nurse training and prior to my Registered Nurse training. The course took place in London during the period of 1980 – 1981 and up until moving to Reading for the Registered Nurse course in 1982.

I trained as both a State Enrolled Nurse and a Registered General Nurse, and experiences of both courses were intermingled and covered in the first book of this series, *Hurry up Nurse: Memoirs of nurse training in the 1970s*.

The procedures and practices outlined throughout this book are a true recollection of my memories of them. I have tried to recreate the events, localities and conversations from my memory and from notes taken at the time, although I have changed the names of individuals and places to protect the confidentiality of patients and the anonymity of others. I have also mixed up identifying characteristics to further protect anonymity. I have changed details relating to the timing of incidents and places and wards where they occurred along with the order of training in some instances.

Moving to London in 1980 proved to be one of the defining moments of my life both in terms of professional and personal development. I made some lifelong friends while working at the London Chest Hospital, and I was supported by two wonderful tutors to go on and further develop my career.

I proudly present this book to the reader and I hope that it will provide you with an insight into hospital life at the time I have written about. London in the early 1980s was a fabulous place to live as many new and innovative treatments were being developed.

# Chapter 1

# London Calling

I took one last look at my beloved bedsit in Leicester, partly to check I hadn't left anything behind and partly to say goodbye. It seemed silly being attached to a one-room bedsit, but I had spent two very happy years living there and was feeling irrationally attached to it at that moment.

Finally I sighed, whispered farewell, and looked at my rather large suitcase containing all my worldly possessions. It was an old brown suitcase that my mum had given me the week before when I had gone to say goodbye. A solid suitcase with two fastening clasps made of metal, a case that was of a type common in the 1970s. My mum had looked a little forlorn as I left, and I tried to make as light of it as possible, promising I would take care of myself and that I would visit when I could. London was only one hundred miles from Leicester but it may have been John o' Groats as far as my mum was concerned.

'Don't worry mam, I'll be fine and I will write and let you know how I'm doing.' Mum was doing her best not to show the sadness she was feeling and smiled as I left, but I knew she would cry when she went back inside the house.

It didn't pay to dwell on these morose thoughts though, and so I locked the bedsit door and dragged the suitcase down the stairs, sneaking past Casanova's flat on the ground floor and stepping outside into the fresh air. Casanova was a man in his mid-forties who constantly had women going in and out of his room at all times of day and night.

It was a bitterly cold Sunday morning in October 1980. I realised I wasn't dressed for the weather, as I had on a pair of light trousers and my favourite beige jacket; I immediately felt the icy cold wind blowing through my jacket and light silk blouse. *Oh well, too late now,* I thought, as all my clothes were in the suitcase and there was no way I was going to try opening it again after sitting on it that morning to make the clasps fasten. It had ended up being a battle of wills between me and the suitcase: I had finished up lying on it and getting it into a judo hold before finally managing to get one clasp to click into place. That had been followed by another monumental effort to get the other one closed. After shutting the front door leading into the house of bedsits that had been my home, I left my suitcase on the doorstep and popped down the road to post my keys through the landlord's door like he had asked me to.

I realised when walking back up the road how quiet it was on a Sunday morning. I looked across the road to the Charles Frears School of Nursing, the magnificent Tudor building where I had trained, and felt another sense of nostalgia. I arrived back at the house and half-carried, half-dragged the suitcase up the road to the bus stop. Thankfully, my bedsit had been fairly close to the main London Road and I crossed over with relative ease, as there was hardly any traffic around. By the time I got to the bus stop I was feeling a lot warmer due to the weight of my suitcase. For the first time that morning I was feeling excited about the adventure ahead of me and couldn't wait to get to London.

I had applied to do a course in cardio-thoracic nursing and had been accepted on the same day as the interview, much to my surprise. I had applied for it a bit late in the August of 1980 when my friend, who was training at Great Ormond Street, had spotted the advert in the Nursing Times. Brenda and I had met while she was doing her adult placement in Leicester during the previous year and we had become great friends. I missed her when she went back to London and she had missed me too, it seemed, as she was constantly on the lookout for jobs that might interest me.

Finally the bus came, just as I was about to cool down again, and I arrived at Leicester train station in plenty of time to catch a train. I had left early, knowing that Sunday buses were few and far between. There were a few more people around by the time I got to the station, and I bought a one-way ticket to London. I had about an hour to kill before my train would arrive and I decided to buy a cup of coffee. The train station was freezing and there was nowhere warm to sit, so I sat trying to think warm thoughts. One of my friends had always said that if you thought of a lovely warm coal fire when it was cold that you would feel warm. I wrapped my hands around the plastic cup of coffee, which was lukewarm due to the cold, and tried this tactic unsuccessfully. I thought back to the interview that I had attended in August when it had been a much warmer day than this one, and a weekday.

I had travelled down to London by train on my day off from the Groby Road Hospital where I had worked after qualifying. I had left at around eight o'clock in the morning despite my interview time being two o'clock in the afternoon. I knew it would take some time to find my way to the hospital by Underground tube train, and I thought I could take a look around the area before going for interview. I was disappointed that Brenda had not been able to get the day off, but she was on an early and we were going to meet in Holborn later that afternoon. The tube had not been too difficult to negotiate and I had sauntered along, arriving at Bethnal Green tube station at around midday. I asked someone in the street how to get to the London Chest Hospital and had been given directions. It was only about five minutes away from the tube station. On turning into Bonner Road, the hospital was the first building I saw, set back on a corner, with metal fencing all around set on a dwarf wall. The hospital itself, though large, was tiny in comparison to Leicester Royal Infirmary. It was probably a similar size to Groby Road Hospital but much more compact, as Groby Road was spread out over a large area of land; however this one had a pleasant look to it. The streets around the hospital left a lot to be desired though, and the area looked generally run down.

I had walked around for quite a while until I realised that it was nearly time for my interview, and then I braved the walk through the hospital gates. The entrance consisted of two very old and foreboding oak-wood doors that were closed shut. I opened one of the big, heavy doors and walked in. I almost fell in, actually, as it opened a lot more easily than I thought it would. I gathered myself together, hoping no one had noticed this, and saw that the hospital reception desk was just inside. The receptionist was on the telephone and I waited while she put various calls through to various wards. She looked at me and smiled. 'Yes?' she enquired.

'I'm here for an interview.' She smiled again.

'Name?' *Obviously she saved her longer conversations for the telephone*, I thought.

'Dawn Brookes.'

'Take a seat.' She nodded in the direction of a bench on the opposite side of the corridor and I went and sat down. I saw her pick up the phone and heard my name mentioned as she spoke. I was around ten minutes early. I couldn't see much of the hospital from here, just a long, marble corridor, heading in both directions from where I sat, which appeared to run the length of the hospital. There was a lot of hustle and bustle, phones ringing, voices everywhere, some laughing, and some shouting. It must have been visiting time, because there were a lot of people dressed in ordinary clothes milling around, some people stopped at the reception desk to ask the way to a ward. I was starting to feel nervous tension, as even though I hadn't got my heart set on the job, the prospect of being interviewed was still nerve-wracking. I heard my name; it was the receptionist.

'Miss Brookes! Left along the corridor, past the stairs, then second door on the left. There's a sign on the door saying "Senior Nursing Officer".'

I got up and walked along the corridor. I found the door but didn't know whether I should knock or wait outside. I was staring at the door like an idiot when it opened and a kindly, Caribbean-looking lady wearing a navy blue uniform opened it. 'We were beginning to think you had got lost,' she smiled. I knew I would like her immediately. 'Come in,' she continued. She wore a lovely frilly hat and for a moment I was fixated with this, but then pulled myself together.

I saw three other people in the room as I entered. 'This is Miss Bale, Senior Nursing Officer, Mr Robinson, tutor, and Mrs Chang, tutor. I am Mrs Lumumba, nursing officer. Sit down, Nurse Brookes.'

They asked me for my certificates and qualifications, and I handed over my enrolled nurse certificate confirming that I was a real nurse and my school certificates, for what they were worth. I had a few CSEs, one O level and not much else. CSE stood for Certificate of Secondary Education and a grade 1 was equivalent to an O level, grade C. Many secondary schools in England, Wales and Northern Ireland only offered CSE subjects to pupils, although some did offer O level subjects to the more academically able. CSEs meant that pupils did at least leave school with nationally recognised qualifications. Both of these examinations were replaced by GCSEs in 1988. Mr Robinson raised a quizzical eyebrow on inspecting the school certificates. I couldn't remember a lot about the interview except for two questions. The first came from Mr Robinson. 'You don't appear to have many school qualifications; why is that?'

I was a bit taken aback, and I felt my face redden as I wracked my brains for an answer. Eventually I explained that I had found school difficult and had experienced some problems at home. They seemed to accept this, and Mr Robinson smiled. He was dressed in a suit, wore glasses and had thin grey hair; he appeared to be in his sixties. He had a lovely twinkle in his eye when he smiled.

The next question came from the lady who had let me in, Mrs Lumumba. 'Tell me a story that shows me how you can deal with stress. It doesn't have to be work-related.'

*Where were these questions coming from?* I saw that all of their eyes were on me. Although the question put me on the spot a bit, I told them how I had been interviewed for the Samaritans a year before and had been asked what I would do if presented with a 'flasher'. A flasher referred to a person (usually male) who would expose themselves in front of others. I related the story to them and then said that I had answered, 'I would say: never mind, perhaps it will grow.' At this they all laughed, and I felt relaxed for the first time since entering the room. That answer was either going to make or break me, but I couldn't think of anything else at the time.

There had also been the customary, 'Why do you want to work here, Nurse Brookes?' question of course, and I had practiced my answer on the train.

'I am really interested in cardio-thoracic nursing, having worked on a medical ward for the past ten months.' As per my first entry into nursing, when asked this question the reality was a bit different to the answer I gave at interview. The real answer should have been, *because my friend has been nagging me to move to London for ages*, but of course I was never going to say that. The interview ended and they explained that the course was due to start in October, and that I was a bit late applying for this year. They asked me to sit outside, which I duly did, except there were no chairs, so I stood. After about twenty minutes they called me back in. They were all smiling.

'Congratulations,' said Miss Bale, 'you have been accepted. You can start in October this year as we have had someone pull out. We will put a letter in the post.' I was stunned. I hadn't expected to be told on the day and I certainly hadn't expected to be moving to London in a couple of months. I had been applying for the following year. *How was I going to tell my mum and how was I going to tell Special?* Special was the ward sister I was currently working for on a medical and infectious disease ward. I had nicknamed her Special because underneath a formidable exterior, I had discovered that she really was quite special. Obviously I never called her Special to her face. I had become fond of her and in spite of her frosty exterior, the feeling was reciprocated. I wouldn't go so far as to say we were like family – she was a bit like the maiden aunt in David Copperfield, and I admired her.

I floated out of the hospital and made my way back to the tube station. Later that day I celebrated with Brenda, who was delighted that it would all be happening so soon, and then I got a late train back to Leicester as I was working the next day.

I received the promised letter in the post the following week. The offer explained that I had been accepted for a twelve-month, fully funded course in cardio-thoracic nursing and told me the salary (the usual pittance) – and there was something mentioned about a London Weighting Allowance that meant nothing to me. I later discovered that the London Weighting Allowance was an extra amount paid to people of certain professions (usually in the public sector but not exclusively), who were employed in London due to the higher costs involved in living there. I was instructed to report to the London Chest Hospital, main reception, on a certain Sunday in October 1980, and I would be given a room in the nurses' home. Enclosed was a health questionnaire for me to complete and return, and I was informed that I would be examined by a doctor during the first week of training.

So, here I was at the station in Leicester at the start of my journey. The train was on time and the journey to London, King's Cross, took about two and a half hours. It should have been much shorter but Sunday trains were always slower, I was informed by the guard who came to check my ticket.

'When will we arrive in London?' I asked.

'Twelve-thirty, duck. Train stops at every station today – its Sunday, duck.'

He must have been from Leicester as the customary 'duck' was native slang to the area. When the train finally arrived in London I realised I was hungry: I remembered I hadn't had breakfast, partly because I'd had no food left in the house and partly due to the combination of excitement and nervousness of that morning. I hadn't eaten on the train because food was too expensive on trains and I was nearly broke already, even though I had been paid in September. Travel, cigarettes and parties had taken most of my salary, and I had spent almost all of my remaining money on the train fare. October was going to be difficult in terms of money but at least I would have a roof over my head. Payment for that would come out of my salary, which would be paid in arrears. I could go into my overdraft if necessary, but that had become more and more common recently. I might have to do some agency work around my new job, I thought.

I heaved my suitcase off the train and realised I was at the far end of the platform; it seemed to take an eternity to get to the ticket barrier, as I had to keep stopping to put the case down and then starting again. I finally made it, and the man took my ticket from me. I dragged the suitcase across the station and arrived at the tube sign. The steps down to the Underground had been a lot easier on my interview day when I hadn't had the heavy burden that I was carrying today. *Never mind*, I thought, *almost there.* I bought a tube ticket and descended the last bit of the way on a wooden stepped escalator. The Underground was busy but not crowded; I could hear a variety of languages as tourists were present even on a cold day in October. There was a busker playing the guitar and singing as I walked towards the platform I was heading for. I smiled at him, but he didn't smile back as I didn't give him any money! I looked at his cap laid on the ground and thought to myself that there wasn't much money in it. If there had been, I might have been tempted to ask him for a loan. The Underground platform was quite busy, as

King's Cross was a mainline station from the north and the midlands into London.

Finally a tube train arrived, and I dragged the suitcase onto it. I was really tired by now and my stomach was rumbling. I had fallen out with my suitcase and kicked it in place as I sat down, but the kick hurt me more than it hurt the suitcase. The train became less and less busy as it headed towards the East End of London. By the time I arrived at Bethnal Green Tube Station there were only three passengers left in the carriage. I had wondered whether I might meet anyone else moving into the nurses' home, but didn't see anyone fighting with luggage.

I got off the train at Bethnal Green and saw to my dismay that the escalator wasn't working. I had to drag that wretched case up hundreds of steps to get out into the daylight. By the time I got to the top I was wondering if my worldly goods were worth this effort, but decided that they were. I did think that I should have left my books behind, as they were probably weighing me down. I had left my cherished Panasonic music centre with my mum and had said I would collect it, along with my records, at the first opportunity.

The final part of the journey seemed to take the longest. I was hungry and thirsty, and my right arm felt like it was going to drop off. In fact, both arms were aching as I had been swapping hands every few minutes. I mainly dragged the suitcase along the pavement now, making a lot of noise as I made my way through the streets to the hospital, but I was past caring. I turned into Bonner Road and saw the welcome gates to the hospital. With a sudden burst of energy, I made my way to the front entrance and then cursed as I saw the steps up to the front doors. They had of course been there on the day of my interview, but I hadn't been tired that day. I sat on the bottom step for a few minutes and smoked a cigarette. Later, in 1983, I gave up smoking. Feeling reinvigorated, I dragged the case up the steps and pushed open one of the big brown doors. *Hello world, I have arrived.*

On entering the hospital I showed my letter to the receptionist, a man this time.

'Hello love, you need to go down the corridor, past the stairs and you'll see doors on the right that take you out into a courtyard. Go straight across the yard and the door to the nurses' home will be right in front of you.' He smiled, then looked at a list in front of him. 'You're on the first floor, right at the top of the stairs, end room on the left, and your name will be on the door.'

# Chapter 2

# Nurses' Home

I found my room at one end of the corridor on the first floor and pushed the door open. The key was in the door, and there was the label with my name on it on the outside. I was a bit disappointed, as the room was tiny compared to my bedsit. As I opened the door it hit the bedside locker, and I looked to the right to see a single bed. At the foot of the bed was a small wardrobe. Against the left-hand wall was a small chest of drawers with three drawers, and there was a sink in the far (well not that far) left-hand corner of the room. The room looked out onto the courtyard and the hospital rear side, and there was scaffolding to the right of the courtyard which was to remain in place for the whole time I lived there.

I sat on the bed, exhausted, and there was a knock on the door, which I had left open. Before I had the chance to reply, in came a very tall, slim girl with dark curly hair. 'Hello,' she said, 'are you starting the course tomorrow?' I detected the Welsh lilted accent immediately.

'Yes, I am, are you?'

'Thank God for that. I've been here all day and haven't seen a soul. My name's Fran, I'm from Swansea.'

'Hi, I'm Dawn, from Leicester. What time did you get here then?'

'My dad dropped me off at ten o'clock. He took me out to lunch and then he had to get back.' *Lunch and a lift*, I thought, *lucky you*.

'I've been travelling most of the day,' I replied. 'Trains are really slow on Sundays and this case weighs a tonne.'

'Do you want a coffee? I've got some welsh cake my mum made too if you would like some,' she offered, and I knew I would like her from that moment on. I nodded enthusiastically. 'I'll be back in a jiffy,' she said, and turned and went away as quickly as she had arrived. The very welcome coffee and cake arrived a short time later, and we both lit up cigarettes and started to share our stories. Fran had trained in Swansea and never lived away from home before, but she said she was up for the challenge.

'I think my parents were beginning to think I would never leave,' she laughed. 'Hints have been dropping for the past two years but now I think they will miss me. They wanted me to marry a boy who lived down the road, not move to London.' Fran was pleasant company after my long journey.

In a while, we started to hear lots of noise and voices as other people arrived. Fran showed me the kitchen that was about halfway along the corridor on the opposite side to my room. It was a good size, with lots of cupboards, a fridge, and a cooker with four gas rings and an oven. There was a kettle and a toaster that both looked like they had seen better days. The bathroom was next to the kitchen and there was a single bath; the toilet was next door to the bathroom. I counted twenty rooms on the floor, and there must have been the same number on the ground floor and second floor. A palace it was not.

A short time later, three other girls had congregated in my room along with Fran. There was May, a vicar's daughter from Bournemouth, Jen from Stornoway (I had no idea where that was) and Blanche, a black girl from Leicester whose parents had brought her down. *If only I had known her before,* I thought. We were soon laughing and joking and sharing life stories, and we became firm friends from that day forwards.

It took a while to get used to Jen's thick Scottish accent but we mastered it soon enough. Stornoway, she explained, was the main town on the Isle of Lewis in the Outer Hebrides. I was no wiser, but have since discovered it is a long way north. It was nice to meet someone smaller than me in Jen; she was four foot eleven inches tall and I was five foot one inch (half inch actually, but I always rounded it up). She had mousy brown hair, similar to mine, although hers was short and mine was shoulder-length. May was medium height with darker brown, shoulder-length, straight hair and a posh accent, and

Blanche was medium height, chubby but not fat, and had a really open and kind face with dark brown eyes and medium frizzy black hair. Blanche was Afro-Caribbean.

'How did you get here?' I asked Jen once I realised that Stornoway was on an island.

'I flew over to Glasgow yesterday and stayed overnight with a cousin, then I got a train to London, but I had three changes before arriving in London. I got a taxi from King's Cross to the nurses' home.' *Blimey,* I thought, *and there was I feeling hard done by.* I related the story of my journey, but it didn't have quite the same impact after hearing about Jen's. May had been driven up by her father and she was looking forward to life outside of a vicarage, she laughed. Blanche was the only one with a steady boyfriend, who lived in Leicester, and she had every intention of moving back there as soon as she had finished the course, as she was already missing him.

By the time we heard people coming off the wards following their shifts we had already gelled into what would become a close group of girls. Fran was the oldest at twenty-three, May was almost twenty-three, Blanche was twenty-two and Jen and I were the babies at twenty-one. At around six o'clock we decided to unpack, and agreed to meet up and go over to the hospital canteen and find some food. I unpacked my suitcase, and was just about to close it when I noticed something in the bottom; it was a letter from my mum with two ten pound notes inside. I was ecstatic; that was a lot of money for me, and maybe I wouldn't have to starve all month after all.

We had found the canteen in the hospital basement and eaten well, as hospital food was relatively cheap, and I think we were all feeling much better as a result. Jen was looking like she might fall asleep at the dining room table.

'Come on girls, I think it's time to call it a night. We need to be in class at nine o'clock in the morning.' May put into words what we were all thinking, so we headed back to our rooms to get ready for the following day. Some of the girls still had to unpack.

I sat down on the bed for a while; there was no chair to sit on so it was the bed or the floor. I looked at my writing pad, thinking that I should write a letter home to my mum. She didn't have a telephone so the only way to keep in touch was to write, and I also wanted to thank her for the twenty pounds which had saved my life. I would miss out telling her that last bit though as I didn't want her to worry; I knew that she didn't have much money herself so I was never going to cadge from her. I had just picked up the writing pad when I heard screaming coming from down the corridor. I opened my door and saw a commotion up near the kitchen, so I went to see what was going on. There was a fair-haired girl standing there, screaming her head off, and a few people had gathered round.

'What on earth's the matter?' I asked.

She just stood there trembling in the corridor. 'In there.' She pointed towards the kitchen. Fran had come out of her room by now, as had May. We looked into the kitchen but couldn't see anything.

'Turn the light off,' the trembling girl said.

Obediently I did what she said and tried to calm her down.

'There, it's off,' I said, beginning to think I had moved into a psychiatric home.

'Now turn it back on.' I did so and as I did, I saw about ten enormous cockroaches crossing the floor before scuttling underneath the kitchen units. We all stepped back, startled, though none of us had quite as dramatic a reaction as the screaming girl.

'That's all we need,' said Fran, who shared that her Nan had a farm in Wales and they were forever invading the kitchen there. At that moment someone popped their head out from one of the rooms down the corridor.

'Would you lot keep it down, I'm on an early in the morning,' she said, and then closed the door.

'Come on,' said Fran, 'you look like you need a nice cup of tea.' She took the trembling girl by the arm and steered her towards her room. May and I followed.

We discovered that trembling girl was called Flora and was also one of our set. I had mixed feelings about having a hysterical girl in the group. She had arrived later than the rest of us as her train had been delayed. Flora was from Hull, and her journey had been rather eventful. First, her dad was going to give her a lift, but he was a vascular surgeon and he had been called into work in the middle of the night, so her mum took her to the train station where she bought her a first class train ticket. *As well for some,* I thought. She had to change trains somewhere along the way and the second train didn't have a first class carriage – *poor thing,* I thought. This train stopped in the middle of nowhere for an hour and nobody knew what was going on. There were very few railway announcements back then, and even if there were you couldn't understand what was being said, and they never told you what was going on. You were lucky if you got: 'This train has been delayed.' The guards were never anywhere to be seen if something was wrong. Finally, the train got moving again, but Flora had lost her seat to someone who took it when she went to try and find out what was happening. Flora had to stand for an hour before arriving in London. She hadn't wanted to brave the Underground so she had made her way to the street and was about to get into a taxi when someone nudged her out of the way and jumped in. Poor Flora was by now terrified of London, and waited for a while before another taxi pulled up and brought her to the hospital. She had just found her room and the kitchen, and was going to make herself a bedtime milky drink when the invasion of the cockroaches occurred. It was obvious to the rest of us that Flora was going to need looking after, or she wouldn't survive a week away from her cloistered upbringing.

Once we had all had a cup of tea, Flora finally calmed down. I had thought about telling her that cockroaches were poisonous, but decided she'd had enough traumas for one night. Fran was in Welsh mothering mode.

'Don't you worry, they're filthy creatures but they are more scared of you than you are of them. I'll ask someone if they can get rid of them tomorrow.' May and I looked at her cynically but she gave us both a warning glance, so we nodded knowledgeably.

'Yes, I'm sure someone will re-home them,' May smiled, and I nearly laughed but for another warning shot from Fran.

'Do you think so?' asked Flora.

'Oh yes,' I said. 'No doubt about it. Anyway, I think I'm going to go to bed now – see you in the morning.' May and I left, and when we saw Fran escorting Flora to her room like a mother hen we knew that we would all be in good hands as long as Fran was around. I also made a mental note not to be the first into the kitchen at night!

I thought it perhaps as well that Flora didn't know the history of our new home, or she may never have ended up moving here. My dad had revelled in telling me stories about the place, taking far too much pleasure in relating the more frightening parts of its history. Bethnal Green, in the East End of London, appeared to have had a dubious past. Probably not more so than any other area in the East End, but its associations with the Kray twins and Jack the Ripper made it rather notorious. We discovered that many locals in the surrounding pubs were quite proud of its fame, albeit from less than desirable celebrities.

The Kray twins were gang members who were infamously responsible for a London underworld of crime and violence. Other members of the family were also criminals, and they had lived in Bethnal Green in their early years, a couple of miles away from the hospital. Almost every pub we went into was reputed to have had the twins drink there, so I am not sure whether I ever drank in one that they had truly frequented. It may well have been true, as Bethnal Green has a long history of boxing and the Krays were boxers in their early years. There were often gangland feuds across the East End as a result of the Kray twins' operations. The Krays had long been imprisoned by the time of my move. For many years Bethnal Green was a poor area, and Jack the Ripper reputedly operated towards the western edge of the area and into Whitechapel.

There were also philanthropists operating in and around Bethnal Green. The Quakers and bankers, for instance, who originally brought the dream of a hospital for people with tuberculosis to life. They were responsible for the building of the London Chest Hospital. Quakers still meet on

Old Ford Road, which was the road I walked along whenever I took a tube into London. There was also a Bethnal Green Medical Mission that had been established to help the poor.

Finally, I got back to the room that was going to be my home, with thoughts of cockroaches and criminals whirring round in my mind. It was boiling in there, despite the cold outside. I noticed there was a radiator under the window but there was no way of switching it off, so in spite of the freezing cold outside, I pulled the top sash window down halfway and crawled into bed. At least there was bedding, because I didn't have any of my own. The white, starched sheets were uncomfortable, and as I fell asleep I wondered if they doubled up as hospital sheets – I hoped not, but suspected they might.

# Chapter 3

# School Again!

Crash, bang! I awoke with a start, wondering where on earth I was, and then I remembered. It seemed the girls starting on the early shift weren't too concerned about waking anyone up as they banged around and slammed doors, or maybe they were getting their own back from the night before. The girl in the room next to me must have been on an early, as I could hear her crashing around in her room and the taps running. Every time someone turned on a hot tap the pipes gave off clanging noises, which eventually turned into a high-pitched whine. This was going to take some getting used to, I thought to myself.

I was freezing cold and wondered why, but remembered I had left the window open and it was howling a gale outside. The net curtains were blowing around in the room, and a picture I had put on the window sill was now on the floor. I looked at the clock: six o'clock! I had never been a morning person. I dragged myself out of bed, closed the window and went back to sleep, waking again at eight o'clock when my alarm went off. I was used to sharing a bathroom and toilet from my bedsit days, but every time I went down the corridor to the toilet, it was locked. When I was getting near to bursting point, I decided to go up to the next floor and found the one up there unoccupied. There were three floors to this nurses' home, which was one of three residences. There was a residence for trained staff and one for the doctors who were on call; we were in Residence 2 which was for course trainees. We were all qualified nurses but were training for a specialism, so it was back to being a student for a year.

I decided a strip wash was going to have to do it, and then a cup of coffee. I did at least have a jar of coffee which I had brought with me, but no milk. Fran had said the night before that I could use hers, which she had clearly labelled and put into the fridge – as if that was going to make a difference. I would soon learn that labels meant nothing in a nurses' home, and if you wanted to keep any food for cooking, it was best kept in your own room. Things had a habit of walking, and in spite of the rude messages stuck to the fridge and cupboards, no-one took any notice. There wasn't a lot of room for storage anyway as the shabby cupboards were pretty full and some people had even put their names on the doors. The fridge was large but antiquated, and it certainly wouldn't have passed the CFC emissions tests of today. In fact it was probably this one fridge alone that was responsible for a large proportion of global warming. The bacteria that grew inside it could also have filled a pathology laboratory for biology students who wanted to practice growing stuff in their Petri dishes.

I met Fran and the others downstairs, as we had arranged to congregate at the entrance and go over to the classroom together on our first day. The classrooms were on the ground floor of another residence – the one where permanent staff lived. As we entered, we met the other girls who were going to be in our set. There were ten of us in total.

Mrs Chang entered the room; she was a bundle of energy, small, rotund and always smiling. She spoke as fast as she moved and I knew I would like her. She was nothing like the serious but kindly Mrs Butcher who had been my tutor in Leicester. Mrs Chang had moved to England from Malaysia in 1970 to find work. She was in her early thirties and had married a Malaysian man who she had met whilst working at St. Thomas' hospital in London. She had become a nursing tutor in 1977, the same year I had started my initial nurse training. The room was set out with tables rather than desks, and we all found seats. Mrs Chang began by introducing herself and then, after she had called out our names from a register, she asked us to introduce ourselves and say where we had come from.

Six of us had already met so we were eager to meet the rest of the group. Chloe introduced herself as being from London, and explained that she lived in a flat not too far away in Bethnal Green. She was originally from the West Indies, but her family had moved to England when she was four years old, and she had moved to London to do her general training in 1977. She had studied at Bart's (St. Bartholomew's) hospital for her training and continued there after qualifying. Supindra had been born in England and was still living at home with her family, who were from India; she had worked at The London Hospital in Whitechapel before starting the course. Margaret was from Margate in Kent, and she had moved into the nurses' home, although we hadn't met her the day before. She said that she had arrived in the evening, and had heard the screaming episode while she was unpacking but hadn't come out to investigate because she had been a little bit scared of the noise. Fran and I looked at Flora, who blushed. Kath introduced herself as being from Bristol, but told us she had moved to London a year before and was living with her boyfriend in Hackney.

I could tell immediately that we were going to gel as a group. The only one we didn't get to know quite as well was Kath, but the rest of us became good friends and often socialised together. Kath did join in and was great fun during class and on the wards, but she had a life outside of the hospital.

'Now we have all introduced ourselves, let's get started,' began Mrs Chang. 'As you are aware, the course you are embarking upon is the Joint Board of Clinical Nursing Studies (JBCNS) 162 – cardio-thoracic nursing. It will last twelve months, and you will gain a multitude of experience in this hospital.'

Mrs Chang continued in this vein for a while, explaining that there were two main wards on the second floor of the hospital as well as an intensive care unit for cardiac surgery. The wards on the second floor were called Riviere, which was a medical ward specialising in tuberculosis, and Hilton, which was also a medical ward. On the first floor of the hospital were two surgical theatres, a high dependency chest unit for people post-lung surgery, a surgical ward called Lister, and the coronary care unit. The ground floor of the hospital housed the out-patients department and a cardiac catheter laboratory as well as all the administrative offices, including those of the nursing officers. In the basement were the canteen, the main kitchens, the mortuary and post-mortem room.

'You will rotate through all of these wards (thankfully not the mortuary) and units on both days and nights,' – groan – 'but you will have to go over to the Brompton Hospital for your paediatric experience as we don't see children at this hospital.' Double groan, scary, I thought. Mrs Chang then moved on to explain how the course was assessed, and we were all delighted to know that there would be no final exams but that we would undergo continual assessment. Actually this did involve a lot of hard work, but not having a final exam was a bonus. The continual assessment would involve tests once a month; two case studies, one cardiac and one medical; and successfully passing all ward placements. In addition to this we had some practical skills to pass, including giving intravenous drugs. The latter was one of a number of extended roles for nurses, previously undertaken by doctors that were gradually introduced from the late 1970s onwards.

The scaffolding outside my room, I learned, was to be a hospital extension where another ward and theatre would be added, but this was not completed until after I left the hospital in 1982.

'On this course you will cover respiratory disease, including in-depth anatomy and physiology as well as surgical techniques; and cardiac disease in the same manner.' Mrs Chang obviously loved teaching, she was so enthusiastic. For the first time in my life I was beginning to realise that learning could be fun. There was no formality with Mrs Chang, and – a first for me – we were allowed to call each other by our first names. We did respectfully call her Mrs Chang, but she never made us call her Sister Chang. 'We have recently started to treat lung cancer with cytotoxic drugs (cancer chemotherapy was in its early stages) and we are very excited about this.' Mrs Chang explained that after a coffee break we were to go to the outpatients department to see Dr Caplin for a medical examination.

Dr Caplin was a chest consultant at the London Chest Hospital and specialised in tuberculosis. He was an incredibly intelligent man with a social conscience. Apparently he had been born in the East End after his Jewish parents had fled persecution in Poland during the First World War. He remained committed to the people of the East End throughout his life, and even founded a refuge for homeless people with tuberculosis (TB). He was sixty-three when I met him and had started to specialise in lung cancer and chronic bronchitis. He insisted on meeting all the new trainees and ensuring that we would not become victims to tuberculosis which, although declining, would make resurgence in the East End of London in later years. Dr Caplin earned an OBE in 1983 and had a ward named after him at the London Chest Hospital, which I left in 1982. Sadly he developed dementia in his later life and died in 2011. I knew nothing of all this when I waited outside his room to see this widely renowned man; to me he was just another physician.

'Nurse Brookes.' The nurse called me in.

'Good morning, Nurse,' Dr Caplin looked at me.

'Good morning, Doctor.'

'Have you ever been in contact with TB?'

'Yes Doctor, there was a patient on my last ward who died of the condition.' He raised his brow quizzically and I could see he was genuinely interested.

'Really? What happened?' I explained about the homeless man I had cared for, and about Special (I didn't call her that) telling me that I would never see a chest X-ray like that for the rest of my career. He was even more interested now, and obviously impressed with my previous ward sister.

'Describe the X-ray, Nurse.' I could see the nurse in the room looking at her watch and knew the others would be queuing up outside, but Dr Caplin didn't seem in a hurry, so I described what I had seen. I explained how both lungs on the X-ray had looked like they were full of caseated cheese. He was suitably impressed by now.

'I have certainly seen such X-rays in my time but not recently, so Sister Froome may be right, let's hope you never do see another X-ray like that one – okay Nurse, we had better examine you.'

After listening to my chest and heart, checking my blood-pressure and pulse he looked for the BCG mark on my left arm.

'Sorry Nurse, it's not visible; we are going to need to give you a tine test.' I had been given a BCG, following a negative heaf test at school, and had declared this on my health form before being accepted, but if the scar was not visible Dr Caplin was not going to take any chances.

The heaf test and tine test are multi-puncture tests where four to six needles coated with tuberculin bacilli are pressed onto the skin of the forearm. The heaf test would be read between two and seven days, but the tine test could be read within forty-eight to seventy-two hours and was favoured by Dr Caplin. In the USA the Mantoux test is used and the tine test is not recommended. The heaf test is now discontinued as a test.

Growing up in England in the 1960s all children were given a BCG vaccine to protect against tuberculosis, if showing a negative heaf or tine test in-between the ages of ten and fourteen years. In my school we were given it at fourteen years of age, and I remember having both the heaf test and then the subsequent BCG (Bacillus Calmette–Guérin) vaccine. The vaccine stopped being given routinely in 2005 in the UK. I didn't mind having the tine test, as I too would rather not have developed TB, and the test was no more than a scratch. Thankfully mine was positive a few days later, meaning that I did not have to have a repeat BCG. Even more thankfully, I never developed TB either. As I was leaving Dr Caplin asked, 'Where did you work before, Nurse?' and he wrote the ward and hospital name down. I suspected he wanted to take a look at that X-ray, and Special would be hearing from him.

After our medicals, we had lunch in the canteen and then went back to the classroom.

Three of us had needed a tine test and we had fun looking for each other's BCG scars before Mrs Chang joined us.

That afternoon we began our studies, starting with the respiratory system. Mrs Chang explained that the majority of our teaching would be provided by herself, as our classroom tutor, and Mr Robinson, the kind man I had met at interview. The consultants would also do some teaching, as would their registrars. Registrars were doctors who had worked as junior hospital doctors and had chosen to specialise in an area such as surgery, cardiology or medicine. A lot of our learning would take place on the job, but I was used to that. We had this initial week's block training and then we would have a day a week in class, with a couple of extra blocks towards the end of the course. This was similar to original training, but much more needed to be crammed in this time. The assessments would take the form of written classroom tests, case studies and ward reports.

Unlike Mrs Butcher, who had assured us of dropouts and failures, Mrs Chang promised us that we would all complete the course and that although it would be hard work, we would be very happy at the London Chest Hospital. She was right on both counts. To be fair to Mrs Butcher, the dropout rates in general training are much higher than those for specialist courses, and the numbers starting training are much greater too.

That first week we were immersed in lectures each day, and Mrs Chang managed to make our learning fun, although it was delivered in great depth. We had to learn physiology from the cellular level, particularly if we were to understand what occurs in chronic bronchitis and emphysema. These were the conditions we were to learn first, along with asthma, and we had to understand the physiological changes within the lungs so that we could understand the treatments. At that time there were only two types of inhaler available to treat asthma and these were salbutamol and becotide. Salbutamol could also be given via nebulised oxygen, which was a frequent treatment for acute attacks that resulted in patients being hospitalised.

Salbutamol tablets were commonly given to people with asthma, as were aminophylline injections. The latter is rarely used in current practice and there are a multitude of inhalers on the market now.

I already knew about nebulisers because we had used them on my previous ward. A salbutamol solution was inserted into a chamber attached to an oxygen mask – the oxygen was then turned on and this forced the solution to be dispersed as a spray, which meant the inhalation provided greater relief. The relief was probably more due to the fact that the patient received the correct dose of salbutamol; since due to difficulties with mastering the technique (particularly when the patients struggled to breathe in the first place), most patients hardly got any salbutamol from the inhalers.

As we got used to our daily routine and living in the nurses' home, we started to explore the local area. As previously mentioned, Bethnal Green was not the most salubrious of places. The houses opposite the hospital were, like the hospital, Victorian buildings, and they had grand steps leading up to their entrances. The majority of these had been turned into flats and were not usually lived in by families. Historically they had probably housed quite wealthy people with servants.

The London Chest Hospital site formed a triangle on a plot of land with sides leading onto three streets. The main entrance was accessed through the main gates on the corner of Bonner Road. The hospital had been initially built by the Quakers in the 1850s for people with tuberculosis (then known as consumption), because there was nothing available to treat patients with the condition in the East End of London. Patients were not allowed into ordinary hospitals for fear of spreading the disease. Coincidentally, the architect chosen to design the hospital had originated from Leicester, like me, so I was obviously destined to work there. The hospital had quite a large lawn area to the front. Balconies were added to the wards in the early 1900s. Prince Albert had laid the foundation stone when building had commenced. It wasn't named The London Chest Hospital until 1923, having had two other names prior to that. The hospital had suffered bomb damage during the Second World War, when the chapel and the nurses' home were destroyed, as well as one of the wards. Thankfully no-one died, although some patients and a nurse were injured. During a second bombing raid the pathology laboratory was also destroyed, along with historical records and specimens. It became an NHS Hospital when the NHS was founded in 1948 after the Second World War. The London Chest Hospital was one of the first hospitals to undertake coronary artery bypass surgery in the 1960s.

During that first week we were given our uniforms. I loved the uniform; it was a green dress because I was still an enrolled nurse at this time; I later left the hospital in 1982 to do my registered nurse training. The dress was made of much thicker cotton than the one I had worn in Leicester, but the best was yet to come. We got to wear starched white aprons, just like I had seen in magazines of nurses from the past. Now I felt like a real nurse. Not only were we given aprons but we were also given starched white hats – I felt I was in nursing heaven. These uniforms were so much smarter than the ones worn in Leicester. I couldn't wait to get onto the wards. In addition to this we were given five uniforms each, one for every day of the week; no more fighting with laundry to try to get uniforms washed in time as I had had to do on many occasions while working in Leicester, where we were only given three uniforms. Sometimes I had to wear a uniform two days running, but it wasn't pleasant, as usually there was some blood or other unsightly stain from a previous shift. I had also worn cardboard hats in Leicester, but I had better not get started on that one. These starched linen hats were beautiful in comparison. We were all happy with the uniforms, although some were not quite as enthusiastic. Jen said her uniform in Stornoway was far superior. Jen was a bit homesick so everything in Stornoway was far superior at this point, but she soon settled as we found the local pubs and clubs and started to explore London.

One of the first places my friends and I discovered on that second night was the local pub, called The Bonner. It was actually The Bishop Bonner but it was known locally as The Bonner and that was the name that stuck. The Bonner stood alone on a street with derelict houses. I believe that Chas & Dave used to sing there regularly, but if they did, it was before my time. There was often live entertainment though, both during the week and at weekends. We found the pub after school on that first day and would go there a couple of times a week until we began to explore further afield. It was a busy pub and all the locals used it. We stood out as it was obvious we were not local, but the people were friendly and were used to staff from the hospital popping in for a pint – or a half in our cases.

I was delighted to discover Victoria Park on my second day of living in London: a huge park that our nurses' home backed onto. We could go out of the back gates and be there in minutes. That park would become my refuge, and I would spend hours and hours in the summer months walking and reading there.

The first weekend in London, Jen, Fran, Blanche, May, Margaret, Flora and I decided to go to the cinema in Leicester Square. I don't remember what film we saw that weekend – I think it was pretty boring actually – but I do remember going to see the second Star Wars film later that year. After we had been to the cinema we found a nightclub called the Empire in Leicester Square and agreed to go dancing. It cost a fortune to get in, and although I was twenty-one I was age checked (you only had to be eighteen to get in, but I always looked younger than I was). I hated this, as it happened to me a lot in those days, but of course I am thrilled now that I look so much younger than my years.

We had a great time, drank too much and shared a taxi back to the hospital at three o'clock in the morning, as the tube trains had stopped running. As I fell into bed that night I realised that I couldn't live like this if I wanted to stay solvent, and decided to join an agency as soon as possible to earn some extra cash.

One thing stood out to me following that night out, and that was having our handbags searched when entering public places. The IRA were very active during the 1970s and 1980s and

London was a prime target, hence the need for these searches. They became particularly noticeable when going out the theatre, to a concert and to places like Wimbledon, where I went later on in my training.

That Sunday I hardly saw anything of my friends, as I think we all felt pretty lousy. I woke up with a splitting headache but did manage to sleep through all of the early shift workers getting ready and the door-slamming. The nurses' home was relatively quiet as some people had gone home for the weekend and others were working. Once I had drunk three cups of coffee and eaten some toast (someone else's bread), I told myself that I must get some food basics in and return all the 'borrowed' food I had eaten that week. I decided to go and explore Victoria Park. It was a bright but cold winter's day and I felt pretty happy, looking back on my first week in London. So far, so good. I had met some lovely people and Mrs Chang was dynamite in the classroom, making lectures far from boring. She managed to hold my attention almost all of the time, which was a first in my life. I have to thank her for the love of studying and learning that I have developed throughout the years since then.

I followed the path into the park and after about ten minutes came to a lake. I walked away from the path and closer to the lake area until I found a secluded spot, and noticed a large rock by the shoreline. I found a comfortable position where I could sit and watch the water and the sky, and sat there for quite some time. I would have stayed longer but the cold was starting to bite and I realised I needed to walk some more to warm up. That spot became my refuge during my first year at the hospital, and I called it 'my rock'. I would frequently visit my rock and spend hours thinking and contemplating life there; I would also take books in the warmer weather and go there to read when I wasn't working or at the end of an early shift.

My rock met three of my needs. The first was that I had a love for water and so the lake enabled me to relax, particularly if work had been stressful. The second was my need to think. I was still very young but found that I was a deep thinker and would mull over all sorts of things in my mind. The third was my love of reading; I had always loved books and preferred reading to any other activity, although dancing and parties came a close second. My rock and I were destined to meet each other, and that solitary place in that busy park offered me solace on numerous occasions.

# Chapter 4

# Spit it Out!

Although I was a qualified nurse, this hospital was a specialist centre, and caring for the patients who were admitted was not at all simple. The medical conditions were complex and I was a new girl once again. Starting a new job was always daunting, but having had a week of specialist lectures I realised that this one was going to be quite demanding in terms of both stamina and knowledge. The only textbooks I had, if you could call them that, were my revision books and my Baillières Nurses' Dictionary which every nurse who trained in the 1970s had a copy of. I still have this dog-eared dictionary – it had a front page on which you could put the start and end date of your nurse training, and I must have been feeling conscientious as it is fully completed. It remains a treasured possession.

Thankfully, Mrs Chang gave us a lot of handouts (the paper variety) as I didn't have any spare cash for books; not that there were that many specialist books for nurses back then, though there were plenty for doctors. Come to think of it there were hardly any nurse memoirs written back then either; the only one I had come across was Monica Dickens' *One Pair of Feet* (still a favourite) and she hadn't exactly been a career nurse, as she had moved on to do many different jobs. There were of course biographies of Florence Nightingale, but reading about the Crimean war didn't appeal to me, although I have since read a few biographies about our Flo, as she is known in the profession.

The shifts at the London Chest Hospital were similar to those I had worked previously. The early was 07.30 am to 4.30 pm, the late was 12.30 pm to 9.30 pm and nights were 9 pm to 07.45 am. I had looked at my timetable and seen that my nights would start in the following February, then decided it would be best not to look too far ahead as I had enough to learn in the present.

The second morning after starting on my first ward, I bumped into Fran when leaving the bathroom. I was not a morning person and didn't like undue conversation, especially not at 6 am. I had hardly slept, looking at the clock every hour, as I hadn't wanted to sleep in. Fran was just the opposite; she loved mornings and looked immaculate. Her hair was well groomed and she had a wonderfully upright posture, which is something I have never been able to achieve.

'I'm so excited,' she said with a smile. 'First day on CCU.' (Short for coronary care unit.) 'I went to the ward yesterday to introduce myself and they all seemed very friendly.' *Why hadn't I thought to do that before my first shift yesterday?*

'That's great, can't wait to hear about it later,' I mumbled, as I walked back to my room. I felt a little better once I had dressed into my uniform. At least I only had to walk across the courtyard and up two flights of stairs to get to work, rather than take two buses like I had done previously. That cheered me as I ate a slice of toast, finished my coffee and smoked a cigarette before making my way over. Blanche was going to be working on the same ward as me but she was starting the next day. She had been given the Monday and Tuesday as days off. I was off later in the week, but we would be working together at the weekend.

My first ward was one of the medical wards and it was named Riviere. I'm not quite sure where the name came from, but it seemed a bit of an odd one for a hospital ward. The ward was for people with respiratory problems and also housed patients with tuberculosis. The wards were not Nightingale wards such as those I had been used to in Leicester. They were accessed up two flights of cantilever stairs (I loved those stairs) with metal railings. Once you got to the second floor there were two huge archways that separated them, Riviere to the left and Hilton to the right.

There were statues carved into the archways all around the hospital. There was even a statuette of Jesus over the main entrance to the hospital. 'This must have been what had attracted the God squad,' I used to joke to my friends. My friends and I had heard that there was a group of Christians working at the hospital, collectively known as the God squad – more on that later in a later chapter. In reality it was not uncommon for Victorian buildings to have statues carved into pillars and the architect (from Leicester) had previously designed churches.

The wards were divided up into bays, with a day room on each floor. There were small toilets in the centre for patients who were too ill to get to the main bathrooms at either end. The ward kitchens were also in the centre of each floor. There was a Sister's office at the far end of each ward and this is where we would have handovers.

The handover was given by a senior nurse on one shift to the nurses coming onto the next shift. There were usually three handovers in any given day. The staff working on an early shift were given a handover from the nurse in charge of the night shift. Staff on the late were given a handover by the nurse in charge of the early, and then the night staff were given a handover by the nurse in charge of the late shift. Every patient would be discussed, along with any important information such as when drips were due, what medications had been changed, how often 'obs' were required, any changes in their condition, any new results and diagnoses, visitors they had seen, what mood they were in and so on. We would dutifully write everything down on scraps of paper and refer to these throughout our shift. At the end of a handover we would be allocated our work by the nurse in charge and then we would disperse. The two nurses in charge would stay and chat for a bit longer, probably sharing the latest gossip while we got on with the work.

There are many things that stood out to me when I first started working at the London Chest Hospital. The first was that there were no student nurses, just post-qualified nurses like myself undertaking specialist training. We inevitably became the students, although not to quite the same extent as during general training. For the most part we were treated with a little more respect, although there were still a few dragons who felt it was their right to tread us underfoot like unwanted ants.

There were of course nursing auxiliaries, who, as always, were the backbone of the hospital wards. They could make or break a ward and they often knew quite a lot more than they were given credit for. After all, some of them had worked at the hospital long before many of the trained staff; even the ward sisters were relatively new to the hospital. There were no Specials at this hospital. Special was a sister who had worked on the same ward for the majority of her career, but London hospitals tended to have a more fluid workforce. Often this was due to the costs of living in the big city, which even back then was expensive compared to the rest of the country. This became apparent as I discovered that most of the trained staff lived in hospital accommodation or rented flats in the East End of London.

The next thing that stands out in my memory is the sputum rounds. I had noticed the sputum pots at the bedsides on my first day. Sputum, as eloquently defined in my Baillières Nurses' Dictionary, is:

*'Excess of secretions from the air passages. It consists chiefly of mucus and saliva, but in diseased conditions of the air-passages it may be purulent, blood-stained, frothy, and contain many bacteria.'*

The dictionary follows this definition with a warning:

*'Sputum should always be regarded as highly infectious and should be expectorated wherever possible into disposable containers and incinerated.'*

Many patients ignored that latter part as they insisted on swallowing the sputum. In lectures we had learned all about the multitude of things that could be discovered from sputum. That may be the case, I thought, but unfortunately there were no students to delegate the daily checking of sputum to, so this was left to the trainees, much to our displeasure. It was something I never got used to; it didn't matter how many times I carried out this routine, my stomach would always retch. I think that particular job was responsible for my life-long stomach problems.

As we were working in a chest hospital and the two wards on the second floor were designated chest (respiratory) wards, in strict obedience to my revered dictionary, every patient had a sputum pot on a locker at the side of their bed. These were white plastic containers not dissimilar to those that used to be used in fish and chip shops, hence my dislike of mushy peas in a pot. They did have lids, and the patient's name was written on the lid along with the date, since they had to be changed every morning and replaced with new ones. Early shifts therefore involved lifting the lid and examining the sputum as well as estimating the amount.

'When you check sputum,' Mrs Chang had taught us – I would have preferred that to be an 'if' – 'you are looking at colour, consistency and amount. The colour will tell you if there are signs of infection; you also need to check for blood, and if blood is present you need to assess the colour, type and consistency of that too.'

I remember there had been lots of cries of 'yuck!' from that class. We had learned that clear sputum meant no infection but large volumes of clear, frothy sputum might indicate pulmonary oedema, where there was fluid on the lungs as a result of heart disease. Yellow sputum was typical of chronic bronchitis and emphysema, while green sputum was usually a sign of infection or chronic infection in patients with bronchiectasis or cystic fibrosis. Blood in the sputum could be from pneumonia, lung cancer, tuberculosis or pulmonary embolism. I would come across patients with all of these conditions and more at some stage during the next year.

'I'm not sure I will be able to examine sputum Mrs Chang. Can we opt out?' Blanche had asked. Mrs Chang had laughed, thinking that Blanche was joking, but most of us were feeling much the same. It was one thing collecting the occasional sputum sample to send off to the laboratory; it was quite another to examine the stuff in detail.

'I will tell the patients it's best for them to swallow it,' whispered Jen.

'You wouldn't!' exclaimed Fran. Jen smiled in response and we weren't sure whether she was kidding or not. Fran was about to say something else when Flora piped up.

'Oh, I'm not worried about it at all.' Flora surprised us with this flippant comment after the cockroach fiasco of the night before. Jen looked at her disbelievingly.

'My cousin has cystic fibrosis,' she explained, which made us all nod understandingly. I resisted the temptation to suggest that some sputum might look like mashed cockroaches but giggled to myself at the thought.

Graham was the first person I met with a diagnosis of cystic fibrosis, which was a condition I had not come across before – mainly because patients with the condition were seen by specialist hospitals such as this one. Graham was sixteen years old and a regular in-patient to one of the wards, with frequent infections. He had blond hair and blue eyes, was around five feet five inches tall and apart from being very thin, pale and barrel-chested he could have been an ordinary sixteen-year-old. Cystic fibrosis was, and still is (albeit with a much better prognosis), a life-limiting condition that babies are born with. The condition is not always obvious at birth and there is now a screening programme to detect it in newborns. Most patients with the condition would die in their teens or early twenties and never reach adulthood. Nowadays people survive well into their forties, and this is likely to improve even more in the future.

Cystic fibrosis cannot be caught, as it is a genetic disorder. The gene is carried by the parents, and when two people who carry the gene marry, there is a one in four chance that a child will be born with the condition, and a two in four chance of a child being a carrier of the defective gene. The condition mainly affects the lungs, causing thick mucus and sputum, which has to be expectorated frequently to limit the number of chest infections a person suffers. It also affects the digestive system, meaning that the patient has to take enzyme supplements to help with digestion. Men with cystic fibrosis are also infertile, which has become more of an issue in recent years as people with it now live longer. Men with healthy sperm can now father children through the aid of fertility clinics. Women with the condition can usually have children, although some may need fertility treatment.

By the time I met Graham he understood better than I did how to manage and treat his condition. Every morning he and another boy called Dave would treat themselves with postural drainage, and then we would give them physiotherapy to try to keep the lungs clear. Postural drainage involved elevating the bottom part of their bodies so that their chests were lower than their legs, and the use of gravity would help them to cough up the sputum. I met a wonderful, cheery, Chinese physiotherapist called Bart who taught me this procedure and the physiotherapy required.

'You need to 'cup' your hands and then tap very quickly from the base of the lungs to the top, like playing the drums,' Bart smiled. I was far too gentle when I started out but I didn't want to leave these very thin boys with chest bruises to add to their problems. Bart was a patient teacher.

'Nooooo,' he would laugh. 'Show her, Graham.' With that, Graham would tap himself with one hand and was far rougher that I would ever be.

'Okay, let me try again,' I smiled, and gradually with help from the physiotherapist and patients I learned the technique, which I remember to this day.

Over the next two years I got to know Graham and Dave quite well, as they were frequent visitors to the hospital both as inpatient and outpatients. Graham sometimes joined us at the local pub when he was undergoing treatment, and I met him for a day out in Hampstead Heath, near to where he lived, the following spring. I don't think I ever saw Graham low in mood although he had every reason to suffer with mental health problems. He was amazingly well balanced and resigned to living a much shorter life than the majority. I found it difficult to understand how he could be so positive but he just was. I grew really fond of him and Dave and would have found it very difficult if either of them had died while I was working at the hospital.

There were times when one or other of them was admitted in a really bad way when they had chest infections. Seeing them struggle to breathe was heart-wrenching. We used to open the windows on the ward to encourage air flow, give them nebulisers, and they would start intravenous antibiotics. The worst time for them was evening and night as the stickiness in the lungs got worse in spite of hourly postural drainage and physiotherapy. Their beds would be placed on wooden blocks to tilt the head down so that the sputum could come up. After a day or two they would start to improve and we would see them laugh again, and the light would return to their eyes. I knew, and more importantly, they knew, that one day the treatment would no longer work and they would likely die from one of these infections. Neither of the boys had a girlfriend, and they had both missed so much school time that they had left at sixteen.

Graham's mum had given him some home schooling, more out of necessity than desire, and both his parents had done their best to provide him with as normal a life as possible. He regularly played football with his dad, just kicking a ball around really, because he couldn't run. He loved walking though, as I discovered on my day out with him to Hampstead Heath, and he also loved nature. He told me that if he hadn't had cystic fibrosis he would have loved to work with nature in some way, but his illness meant that he couldn't get a job, because he would have to take too much time off sick. I was impressed with his knowledge: while we were out he could identify birds, spiders and beetles, as well as every type of tree. As a city girl, born and bred, I was suitably impressed because I could only just tell a sparrow from a pigeon. I like to think that when he did die, his parents scattered his ashes somewhere on his beloved Hampstead Heath.

Evenings and nights were tough times to work as most of the patients with acute respiratory conditions couldn't breathe. Mornings were worse for the patients with chronic bronchitis and emphysema as they tried to clear their lungs of the overnight accumulation of sputum. This leads back to the sputum part of the story, which you may have noticed I had to take a break from.

The first morning I was on sputum duty occurred on my second ward day, which was an early. We had by that time been through the sputum lesson with Mrs Chang, and I was asked to check the sputum pots by the ward sister. My stomach heaved at the thought, which was not a good start. I had come across small amounts of sputum on the medical and infectious disease ward I had worked on after qualifying but it was generally collecting a small sample to send to pathology. This was going to be something entirely different. Funnily enough Jen, Fran, May, Blanche, Margaret and I had been discussing the sputum issue in my room the previous night as four of us had been assigned across the two medical wards. Jen and Fran were working on the coronary care unit so they didn't have to face this just yet. The others in the group were allocated to the surgical ward.

'I hate sputum,' I had complained. 'I'm not sure I will be able to check the pots without pulling a face.'

'You'll be fine,' Fran said. 'Don't think about it while you're doing it, pretend it's something else.'

'Like what?' Jen laughed and the conversation had deteriorated from there, none of it very helpful to me.

*Here goes*, I thought, and was greatly relieved to see that the nursing auxiliary was exchanging the used pots for new ones. At that moment Staff Nurse Trenton came up behind me.

'Does that mean I don't need to check them?' I asked hopefully.

'Yes,' replied the staff nurse, 'Kate is a very experienced auxiliary; she will ask you if she's unsure but we decided to let you get used to the ward before dropping you in it.' I was going to love this hospital – no such luxury would have occurred as a student nurse.

'Thanks,' I smiled.

'That's okay. Come on, let's do the 'obs' round.' I followed her to the treatment room where we collected equipment, greatly relieved even though it was only a temporary let off. I would indeed have to get used to pots full of sputum and would have to train my stomach to behave. Once I acquired the ability to assess and estimate amounts of sputum it was much easier, as I could take a cursory glance and immediately notice if there was anything untoward. If not, the lid went back on faster than I could blink an eye and I would move on the next one.

'Obs' rounds, or observations rounds, I was more familiar with. These involved checking temperature, pulse, respirations and blood pressure, and were carried out four- to six-hourly depending on the patient's condition.

There was a bit more to the rounds in this specialist hospital than in my previous experience, particularly in relation to respirations. Many patients with chronic respiratory conditions have faster than normal respiratory and pulse rates, and we had to learn what was normal for a particular patient and what was normal for the condition that they had. This was important, otherwise I would have been forever calling doctors to check up on patients who were actually stable.

In addition to this, patients with such conditions had different levels of breathing, using different muscles, and again it was hard to judge what was serious and what was normal for that patient. Some patients also developed different-shaped chests due to a chronic lung condition. What I thought was going to be a simple 'obs' round turned out to be a real learning experience and I felt inadequate again, like a new girl starting from the beginning, which in some ways was correct. I was half wishing that I had started with the sputum round, but realised that was just plain silly. The round went something like this.

'Staff,' I called.

'Don't worry,' she replied. 'That's a barrel.'

'That's a pigeon.'

'That's a funnel, oh and that's kyphoscoliosis.'

*We'll have a lot to discuss in the pub tonight*, I thought.

I had to call the staff nurse over at least four more times during that first round because, even though I could check the charts and see what the previous respiratory and pulse rates were, I was not always clear that the pattern of breathing I was seeing was normal for the patient. Observations charts were kept on clipboards at the foot of the bed so that they were instantly accessible to nurses and doctors (and nosey visitors). These included charts for TPR and BP, fluid, drugs (medicines), and in some cases additional ones such as IV charts for those having intravenous infusions or intravenous antibiotics.

'Don't worry nurse, Mr Hickson always breathes that way, he is using his accessory muscles to assist due to emphysema,' Staff Nurse had reassured me. Mr Hickson was leaning forward with his elbows on a table, using his shoulders to assist with breathing. This is quite common in patients with emphysema, although we now call the condition chronic obstructive airways disease, or COPD for short. Mr Hickson smiled at me.

'Not to worry Nurse, I'll tell you if I get worse.'

*If you get any worse*, I thought, *you will be dead*. The poor man looked dreadful but was obviously used to breathing with this level of difficulty when in hospital. He looked like he needed more oxygen as he was blue in the face.

'Should I turn the oxygen up, Staff?' I asked.

'No, he's a retainer.' I looked quizzically and she realised I hadn't got a clue what she was talking about.

'He retains carbon dioxide so if you turn the oxygen up it can cause metabolic acidosis.' Again, I looked stupefied. *Where was Mrs Chang when I needed her?* 'He could die,' she said – ah, now that I did understand. Though I thought a little more study was going to be necessary. Throughout that first week I was bombarded with respiratory jargon, most of which I did not understand. Medical jargon would fill volumes of books all by itself. The terminology alone was confusing, without the additional acronyms and made up words.

In my early training we had often used mnemonics to learn anatomy such as when we had to learn the twelve cranial nerves. The only thing was that after a while, we could remember the phrase and the names but could not always the order of the nerves – it was better than nothing though. The mnemonic for cranial nerves was *'On Old Olympus Towering Top A Fox And Gibbon Vaulted And Hopped.'* The difficulty arose because there were so many beginning with 'O' and 'A'. It was a matter of repetition and we did have great fun with this, and many others. Some of the mnemonics would be too rude to mention.

Going back to Mr Hickson, doctors would check his blood gases each day to measure the levels of oxygen and carbon dioxide in his blood as well as the PH. This was before the days of pulse oximeters, which are now used in all hospitals, and there are miniature versions for use in the community. These devices, often referred to as sats monitors, measure the oxygen saturation, and they just clip on to the end of a finger. Blood gases may still be required though when oxygen saturation is low. Blood gases can now be tested from a capillary blood sample through a small nick to the ear, but can also involve the same procedure as used in 1980 where an arterial blood sample is taken. The first time I witnessed the procedure it seemed a bit barbaric, but Mr Hickson didn't seem to mind it at all and said it wasn't painful unless the doctor missed the artery.

'Nurse, I need to check blood gases on Mr Hickson; can you assist?' Dr Graham was a white South African doctor who always spoke in short, clipped tones. I didn't take to him at all, which was unusual as I always tried to get on with everyone. There was something about his manner that I didn't like; he always gave off an air of superiority although he was a junior doctor. Many doctors had a superior attitude but there was something totally unpleasant about him. He was a tall man with curly, light brown hair that looked as though it had been permed. His whole demeanour was condescending, and he was racist. I only discovered this later in the year when he wouldn't allow Blanche to accompany him to carry out a procedure. He said he was too busy, but it was obvious to me that it was because she was black. I had met people who were racist before but never one who was so obnoxious to work with. I was more angry than Blanche over the issue but she shrugged her shoulders and said it was his South African upbringing, as Apartheid was still prevalent in that country. He was pretty horrible to all of us female nurses too so I don't think his prejudice was just restricted to colour. *I dread to think what he'd be like as a consultant*, I thought, as I followed him and closed the curtains around Mr Hickson's bed.

'Hold the wrist, Nurse,' he commanded. *Talk about stating the obvious,* I thought, as I did as instructed and smiled at Mr Hickson. I had to hold the arm out so that the wrist was exposed, as the needle would be inserted into the radial artery where the radial pulse could be felt. The needle was inserted at a ninety degree angle, and I was fascinated to see that the colour of the blood was so bright compared to that of venous blood, which I was much more used to seeing. I realised it would be pointless to ask the doctor any questions as he was clearly disinterested. At the end of the procedure, Dr Graham took the sample and just walked off without a word. I applied pressure to the insertion mark.

'Full of the joys of spring, that one,' said Mr Hickson, as he put his oxygen mask back on. I smiled at him but didn't say anything as I didn't want to let on that I thought the same thing. Professional courtesy was everything back then, and even if we detested a doctor or a colleague, we tried not to be negative in front of patients. At times I am sure this was misguided.

'Let's see if the bleeding has stopped,' I said, and removed the swab I had been pressing. It had stopped and I applied some tape over a clean cotton wool swab that I had placed over the needle mark. 'There, good as new,' I said. 'Do you need anything?' I asked, before leaving him.

'Just a new pair of lungs, Nurse,' he smiled, but there was a faraway look in his eyes as he said it. *If only I could,* I thought sadly, as I smiled and walked away.

As an addendum to this part of my story, I have met and worked with many doctors, nurses and other health professionals from South Africa and none of them have been like Dr Graham. Thankfully he was a 'one off'.

# Chapter 5

# Class Down

One of the downsides to being a nurse, particularly in the early days, is that when you move hospitals or wards you come across new bugs. This often meant that shortly after starting a new job, and particularly in the winter months, our immune systems were bombarded with new strains of viruses and bacteria that we hadn't formed a resistance to. This was particularly true on starting at the London Chest Hospital, and obviously those of us on the respiratory wards where patients were coughing all day long were particularly susceptible. It was in January 1981 that we all started to go down with one thing or another, mostly respiratory illnesses. Those working on the cardiac wards didn't escape though, because we met up for a class once a week, and also the majority of us were in and out of each other's rooms and socialising at night.

Jen was first to go down with a cold that spread to her chest, and she ended up with a chest infection. Of course this brought out the 'fresh air of Stornoway' nostalgia. Jen had actually trained in Glasgow but she was a Stornoway girl through and through. She was off sick and Fran, Blanche, May, Margaret, Flora and I took turns to make sure she was fed and watered. Flora did this with a little less gusto than the rest of us, saying that she was of a weak constitution and that her parents had told her to stay away from bugs – *working in a chest hospital – oh yes, as if that was going to happen.* I made a mental note to self that Flora's parents were probably living in a parallel universe along with their daughter.

Fran, Margaret and May were the next to go down with heavy colds. They soldiered on for a few days but then May developed an ear infection and Fran and Margaret chest infections. Now there were three of us left in the nurses' home to do the nursing after shifts, although Jen soon joined us as she recovered. Flora was forever finding excuses as to why she couldn't take her turn and I was sorely tempted to drop some cockroaches in her room. A few days later Blanche went down, as did the rest of the girls in our set, even those that lived out. Thankfully Fran and May recovered and helped, while Flora spent most of the time in her room.

'I'm going to kill that girl,' moaned Jen. 'Even when she did look after me, she was in and out like a hare. One day she even wore a mask! Can you believe that?' *Yes I could believe it.*

'Never mind,' I said. 'Almost everyone has had it now and they've nearly all finished their antibiotics, so we can get back to normal soon.'

It was quite tiring, working shifts and then playing nursemaid to one's friends in-between, but we all looked out for each other. Well most of us did, anyway. I was quietly congratulating myself on my strong constitution when I developed a rip-roaring headache while on a late shift just before my days off. That night my temperature rose and I went down with the dreaded heavy cold. It wasn't the cold that was the problem; it seemed that all of us developed secondary bacterial infections – probably due to the amount of bacteria floating around in the hospital wards. I was no different; a few days after developing the cold I had terrible pain over my cheek bones and knew it had gone to my sinuses. My temperature was climbing and the pain in my face got worse and worse. Now the girls were looking after me, apart from Flora, who had taken to her room completely now after her shifts.

A few days later, after forcing myself into work with a red face and worsening pain, I had to make the customary trip to the GP in Bethnal Green. He prescribed antibiotics and signed me off sick for a week. That was in the days before we were granted permission to sign ourselves off sick for seven days. The antibiotics did nothing and the pain got worse. Mrs Chang decided it was time to send me to occupational health. The doctor I saw, examined my face, pressing on my sinuses, and said that he would send me over to the Ear, Nose & Throat (ENT) hospital. A phone call later and I was on a bus over to the hospital with Brenda in tow, as she had come over to visit me that day. The beauty of living in London was that there were teaching hospitals everywhere, all keen to get their hands on patients to practise on, which may or may not have been a good thing.

We traipsed across London on buses and arrived at the ENT hospital, which was called The Royal National Throat, Nose and Ear Hospital. The doctor at the London Chest knew a doctor at the ENT hospital and so he had arranged for me to be seen that day. The hospital was on Gray's Inn Road, King's Cross, and I was tempted to get on a train and go home. I was sure my mum could put some Vicks on my chest and all would be well again, just like when I was a child. With a sigh, I followed Brenda into the hospital. We arrived at the Outpatient Department and I showed my letter from the doctor to the receptionist. The department was heaving with people. I was still feeling dreadful and my face was boiling just above my cheekbones where my facial sinuses were. After about half an hour a nurse called my name.

'Follow me,' she instructed, and I did so. I was led into a room where a doctor sat; he read the letter I had brought along and told me I would need my sinuses drained.

*Really? Is that necessary?* I shouted at him in my imagination – in reality I replied, 'Ok, Doctor.'

He then took two very long, wooden sticks (orange sticks – I have always wondered why they are called that) about the length of barbecue skewers but a bit thicker. I think they were probably about six inches long, really. They had cotton wool wrapped around them about one inch in length at one end. The doctor dipped these sticks into a pot of thick yellow/orange stuff (paste actually) and asked me to tilt my head back. *Oh no, what's he going to do with those things?* I thought. The next thing I knew he inserted one of them up my left nostril and punched it through the membrane at the back of my nose. I was trying really hard not to pass out, thinking they would assume I was a typical nurse baby if I did. He then did the same thing with the other nostril, inserting the second stick until I had two of these things sticking out of my nose. I was feeling light-headed by now.

'There you are,' he said. 'That's done, we just need to give them time to numb you and then you will need to come back for the drainage.'

*You have got to be kidding me! Just when I thought it was all over.* On the way back to the waiting room I asked the nurse, 'What was that yellow stuff?'

'Cocaine,' she said. 'Didn't you know?'

*No I b....... didn't,* I thought. 'No.' I replied.

'You were ever so brave; most people faint,' she said as she left me in the waiting room. *Great – now she tells me. I could have allowed myself to pass out after all.* What I must have looked like, sitting there with these two skewers hanging out of my nose, I don't know. Brenda was chatting away but I wasn't feeling much like talking, I had my head in my hands feeling very sorry for myself. To cheer myself up I decided to explain in graphic detail what had just happened. I was pleased to see that Brenda looked a bit pale too when I related this, but saw that other patients were looking a bit frightened, so I decided to spare them and changed the subject.

Finally the nurse called me again. I took a quick look at the exit and wondered about doing a runner – King's Cross Station was looking very inviting right now. Having second thoughts due to my nasal appendages I turned and followed the nurse sheepishly back to the torture chamber, where Robert the Bruce was waiting gleefully. Was it the cocaine, or did I really see manacles and chains in there?

'Sit down and put your head back, and we'll get on with it,' instructed Robert the Bruce. *This can't be happening,* I thought, as I saw him pick up what looked like a chisel. In fact it was a bone chisel. He removed the orange sticks, which were now orange due to cocaine staining – *give me back my cocaine* I thought as he inserted said chisel into my right nostril. While the nurse held the back of my head he applied incredible pressure and I could hear the bones crushing as he forced the chisel through the bone to allow entrance into the sinus cavity. Finally, he had broken enough bone and he sat back looking a little bit breathless himself after his exertion. Thankfully the cocaine had done its job and there was no pain during the procedure.

'Ok,' said Robert. 'We will now drain the sinuses.' *Might as well,* I thought. He inserted a fine rubber tube through the nose and into the cavity. I was starting to think like a nurse now and developed a bit more interest in the procedure. Next he poured water into the cavity through the tubing until the most horrendous-smelling gunge came pouring back out. Yellow and green foul-smelling pus mixed with water and blood filled a bowl that the nurse held. This procedure was repeated three times until he seemed satisfied he had got the worst of the infection out. Both Robert and I looked exhausted by the time he had finished.

'Right, you now need to take these antibiotics for two weeks and you'll be as right as rain,' he said, giving me a bottle containing Metronidazole.

*Where's the cocaine?* I thought. I was quite pleased Brenda had come with me because I felt a bit peculiar on the bus on the way back and my nose was pouring with blood, which it continued to do for a couple of days afterwards. Brenda insisted I come and stay at her place for the weekend as she was off, and I was grateful to do so. Thankfully, I was in much less pain once the pain in the back of my nose had gone, as the pressure had been released. The antibiotics took effect and I was back at work on the Monday. I had bragging rights for a few weeks that I had definitely had the worst infection, although I think some of them thought I was exaggerating. Trust me, I'm not.

The one person who didn't pick up the virus at all was Flora, of course. I think even Fran would have liked her to have picked up something. Once we were all feeling well again we were a lot more forgiving, and more accepting of Flora's delicate constitution.

Mrs Chang was delighted to have us all back in the classroom on Wednesdays so that we could continue with our studies. Friends had collected handouts for any of us that had missed lectures and we occasionally had group revision sessions either in the nurses' home or at Chloe's, whose flat was a short walk away. Those of us who had taken sick time would need to make it up, either by using holidays or tagging time on at the end of the course, because we needed a one hundred percent attendance record to pass.

I only had one other malady during the year and that was toothache. I woke up one Saturday night, a few weeks after the sinusitis episode, with agonising pain in my tooth that paracetamol couldn't touch. I tried everything, including a hot water bottle, and Fran gave me some cloves the next morning but they didn't help either. Thankfully I wasn't on duty on the Sunday. May came over to my room at lunchtime and said she had asked on the ward, and discovered there was a dental hospital open seven days a week. *Another hospital full of eager students*, I sighed, but I was desperate, and nothing could beat the Robert the Bruce episode. The hospital was in Leicester Square, and Fran came with me because she had a day off. We took the Underground tube from Bethnal Green and found the hospital.

I had been to Leicester Square a couple of times night clubbing, but had never seen the dental hospital before. I must have been blinkered because the building, which is now a hotel, was huge. The last time I had had a tooth removed was as a child when dentists were still putting patients to sleep with gas for extractions. I remember being very sick afterwards and was telling Fran about it. We decided to share dental experiences for a while, but thankfully I was seen quite quickly. A dental student introduced himself and said he would pull the tooth for me. I was pleased to see that he was at least supervised by a trained dentist. Having said that, I would have let anyone pull the tooth out at this point as the pain was excruciating. I was sent for a dental X-ray first, and they agreed that the tooth should come out – perhaps as well or I would have pulled it out myself.

The student was a bit clumsy, and I smiled as I recalled giving my first injection, I think this was probably his first too. He had a little accident and squirted local anaesthetic from the syringe into the back of my throat before finding the right place. After three different injections, during which he was over-generous with the anaesthetic (as my face was still getting numb even after he had pulled the tooth out), he managed to remove the tooth on the third attempt. The dentist supervising him was a saint in comparison to consultants, who would have annihilated the poor young man by now and taken over. At one point I wished the dentist wasn't as patient and would take over. Once finished, totally numb down the whole of the right side of my face and unable to move my tongue, I found Fran in the waiting room. I would have smiled but my mouth wouldn't move. I couldn't thank the dentist but I grunted and nodded to say I was alright, and with that we left the building.

As we were in Leicester Square Fran decided we should walk over to Trafalgar Square, which wasn't too far away, and feed the pigeons. All I wanted to do was sleep, but as she had wasted hours of her day off accompanying me to the dental hospital I didn't feel I could refuse. We walked and she talked, as I was still numb. I did start to get some tingling feeling to parts of my face after we had fed hundreds of pigeons.

Trafalgar Square was always packed with tourists, and people from every nationality would buy bags of bird seed to feed the birds, who were totally fearless. The only thing one had to be careful of was to steer clear of any flying overhead so that you didn't get bird poop on your head. I started to relax as the tiredness wore off, and I got a second wind, and even started to enjoy myself. It was lovely to be pain-free. Eventually, Fran had satisfied her need to feed pigeons and she suggested we head back to the hospital.

Feeding the pigeons at Trafalgar Square was a tradition enjoyed by thousands and immortalised in the film *Mary Poppins*, but birdseed sellers have been banned since 2001 and the London authorities made it a criminal offence to feed them in 2003. There are numerous pigeon deterrents in use, and hawks have been used to drive them away. The reasoning behind the new rules was that the poop was damaging Nelson's Column. Whilst I have every respect for our famous landmarks I do think it's sad that tourists and children are no longer able to have this experience.

When we did get back to the nurses' home that day, and the feeling in my face came back hours later, I was able to eat a light meal and have a wonderful night's sleep before going on a late shift the next day.

# Chapter 6

# The God Squad

Shortly after arriving at the hospital we were all advised to avoid what people termed as the hospital 'God squad'. Apparently there were some members of staff who were overtly Christian, and they were referred to as the God squad or Bible bashers. If anyone ever told me to avoid people for any reason then that was one sure way to ensure that I did the opposite. I was still young and had an enquiring mind, and basically didn't have a problem with what others believed.

I would often hear people say that they would not discuss politics or religion, but I felt this was small-minded and I would discuss both. In fact, I would discuss anything. I had spent many years reading fiction in my childhood and my school reports had always commented on this, recommending that 'Dawn should read more non-fiction.'

*Well, teachers,* I thought, *you would be very proud because since leaving school I have definitely enlarged my reading repertoire.* Part of this was down to my friend, Jill, who had recommended nursing to me in the first place. She was a fan of Erich von Däniken, who believed that the visions in the book of Ezekiel in the Bible were those of aliens who had visited the earth in a spaceship thousands of years ago. I did read the von Däniken books, although I had to wonder why the aliens had not returned. I also read many other books about all sorts of things. I had tried to read the Bible as a child but found it too difficult, and my knowledge of it was limited to knowing the names of the Gospels and the Christmas story.

One of my best friends at school had been a Catholic, and I had once attended mass with her, but giggled all the way through, as it was held in Latin. My friend said she would never take me again as I had embarrassed her. The God squad consisted of two ward sisters, some staff nurses and a couple of hospital porters. The first one I came across was a porter whose name was Martin. The hospital was quite small, so we tended to come across the same people again and again. Martin had long, light brown hair down to his shoulders, and I first noticed him sitting in the hospital canteen reading his Bible. He always sat alone, mainly because people avoided him, describing him as a little bit over the top. He was a good-looking young man in his early twenties. I arrived at the canteen for lunch one day and it was really busy, so as Martin was sitting at a table for four I decided to join him. 'Hi,' I said, as I sat down and put my food on the table. 'I'm Dawn.'

'Martin,' he replied, and he put his Bible down on the table.

'Good book?' I asked.

'THE Good Book, Dawn,' he replied.

'Where do you come from?' I tried a different tack.

'I was born in London. I live in Hackney.'

'I'm new here; how long have you worked here?'

'About six months. I did a maths degree at Oxford but realised that God wanted me to be a hospital porter, and so I am following His calling.'

'He's not very ambitious then!' I tried humour.

'Jesus was a carpenter, Dawn, and he was born in a stable.'

*Sounds like my upbringing,* I thought, but decided that this very serious young man would not respond to humour. 'Do you like being a porter?' I continued.

'Yes. I get to pray for people all day and tell them about God.' *No wonder they avoid you,* I thought, but did manage to get a few sentences in before he moved the conversation back to his being a Christian. I decided that his form of religion was probably a bit too much for me too, and whilst I would have been interested in having a conversation about his beliefs, it was all a bit too intense for my liking. I was beginning to understand why some people preferred to avoid discussing religion – not that this had been a discussion. I saw Jen come into the canteen, but as she was about to do a detour around to my table she saw Martin and turned away. Thankfully he got up to go back to work, so Jen joined me.

'There were no seats,' I laughed.

'I'd rather sit in the park,' she responded. 'I said hello to him one day and he replied, "Hello, Jesus loves you,"' she continued, rolling her eyes. 'Even May avoids him and her dad's a vicar!'

'He seems harmless enough; a bit intense though,' I said, and then we started talking about life on the wards. I told her about the South African Houseman, Dr Graham, and how I found him unpleasant and ignorant.

'There are some weird people working in this hospital,' she said. 'Have you met Mrs Lumumba?'

'Not since my interview; she was on the panel. Why?'

'I'm sure I saw her coming out of her office drunk the other night. She was swaying all over the place and she was still in uniform.'

'Really? Maybe she was off duty but not changed out of uniform.'

'Maybe, but I don't think so.' This was a small hospital, and I soon came to realise that gossip spread like wildfire around the place. Some of the gossip was true and some far from true. We ended the conversation and went back to our respective wards to see what awaited us there.

I had been in London for about four weeks before Brenda and I had the same weekend off. We had arranged that I would go and stay the weekend with her in her flat in Holborn, next to Russell Square tube station. It was a room rather than a flat, I discovered, but about three times the size of mine. There was only a single bed but she had a sleeping bag for me to sleep in on the floor. The building was owned by Great Ormond Street Hospital (GOS) and so the GOS students got to live there. Brenda was now nearing the end of her third year. As her course was a combined adult (SRN) and children (RSCN) course she had to do four years. Her uniform was a beautiful pink and white striped dress, and she also wore a white, starched apron like we did at LCH, but her hat was a frilly one whereas mine was plain. We were thrilled to see each other again and we had lots to catch up on, so I knew that we were in for two late nights before I returned to the nurses' home on Sunday.

Brenda cooked her favourite dish, which was chicken casserole with jacket potatoes. I think it was the only thing she ever cooked because I can't remember any other culinary delights. Not that mine would have been any better, as I lived on takeaways except when I was really poor, and then I would cook spaghetti with tinned tomatoes and grate cheese on top, which was my go-to meal in those days.

'How's it going then?' Brenda asked.

'Loving it.' This was the first chance we had had to have a proper talk, as we worked a fair way away from each other and our shift patterns meant we didn't speak much. It was also hard to communicate by telephone as we only had a public telephone in the main hospital and calls had to come through reception – and although there was a phone in the main building where Brenda lived, it was often engaged.

'Mrs Chang, our tutor, is brilliant: she makes classes really interesting and the hospital is so friendly. The girls in the nurses' home are all nice and I have got to know the ones in my set really well.' I paused for breath and as Brenda didn't reply I continued, 'Guess what, we also have a hospital God squad.'

'Really? How do you know?'

'It's one of the first things I learned after moving into the nurses' home: avoid the God squad, I was told. I have only met one of them so far, a porter called Martin.'

'What's he like?'

'A bit strange, to be honest. Every time you see him he mentions God or Jesus; he doesn't seem to be able to have a normal conversation. I saw him in the grounds the other day. "Hello Martin," I said, "nice day." "My Father made it," he replied. "Thank him for me," I'd said. "Why don't you thank him, Dawn?" And that's how every conversation goes. I wouldn't mind having a discussion with him but he doesn't seem to be on the same planet.'

'I'm a backslidden Christian,' Brenda remarked. I must have looked astonished – I hadn't met any of this type of born-again Christian before and now I seemed to be surrounded by them. 'Don't look so surprised. I met a group of girls when I first moved to London and they were into religion so I went along. They took me to a Billy Graham concert.'

*Is he a pop star I haven't heard of? I must be out of touch,* I thought.

'Who's Billy Graham?' I asked.

'He's a famous American evangelist.'

*Not that famous,* I thought, *and what's an evangelist?* – Obviously religious speak was like hospital speak, with its own lingo. 'Anyway, I stopped going to church when I moved to Leicester and haven't been since.' *Hope that wasn't my influence,* I thought. I suddenly had guilt pangs, but realised I had met Brenda when she had been in Leicester for about six months, so was able to breathe a sigh of relief.

'Well, if you go back, don't get like Martin, because he is a bit too heavenly minded if you ask me.'

'I won't,' she promised, and then we moved on to hearing about the sick children she had been looking after recently at GOS. Now she was more senior she was given a lot of responsibility, and when she described all of the tubes and things that she dealt with I had to imagine the ones I used in micro-fashion. After a late night exchanging hospital stories we finally fell asleep.

The next day Brenda introduced me to a fantastic pancake house not far from where she lived. I had never seen pancakes like it. The menu consisted of nothing but pancakes; there were sweet ones and savoury ones, topped with everything you could think of. The plates were enormous, three times the size of a standard dinner plate. I ordered my favourite, which was plain old pancake with lemon and sugar, while Brenda was a little more adventurous and ordered a pancake with berries and maple syrup. The pancakes were relatively cheap for London and I felt pretty full after eating. The pancake restaurant was still there a few years ago when I visited London, so hopefully it continues to turn out huge pancakes for every taste.

After lunch we got the tube into central London and Oxford Street. I fell in love with Oxford Street straight away. I think we went into every shop, including Selfridges and many of the smaller stores. Brenda bought quite a few clothes, but although I had finally been paid I was wary of spending my money in Oxford Street, as I knew that it wouldn't go far. Brenda was okay because her family were well off and supplemented her income, but I had to live on what I earned plus my overdraft facility, so had to reign myself in sometimes. I had learned quickly that money didn't go very far in London. I chose to spend my money on drink and dancing in those early days until I discovered the theatre and classical music later on. I also had to buy food, and there were no large discounted supermarkets around every corner in 1980.

That night we went to Soho, where food was relatively cheap, for a Chinese meal. The area was a bit shoddy and it was packed with restaurants of all sizes. There were bright lights everywhere and I was absolutely fascinated. We ate in a small, budget restaurant that was packed with people even in early November. The meal was brought to us, or should I say thrown at us, as service wasn't their forte. We were given chopsticks and I had great fun trying to eat rice with them. Brenda was quite good at this as she had lived in London for much longer than me and had been out quite a bit. The rice was served in a small bowl and the other dishes on small plates. The idea was to add small amounts of the food to the rice and eat it with chopsticks, holding the bowl in one hand close to your mouth. There were quite a few Chinese people eating in the restaurant and they were shovelling the food into their mouths at a great pace. One of the waiters who had thrown the food on the table showed me how to hold my chopsticks, and I got the hang of picking up bits of meat, but the rice thing was beyond me. After the meal Brenda ordered Jasmine tea, which came in a large pot and was served in tiny cups. I had never had Jasmine tea but liked it immediately, and from then on, ended a Chinese meal if taken in a restaurant with this drink.

The thing I grew to love about central London was the constant buzz of activity and the fact that there was always something going on. People were always out, day and night. It wasn't like that in the East End where I lived; life there was more akin to what I had been used to in Leicester. But because it was so easy to get into the West End, activity was never far away. How could one not fall in love with this city? Even with the constant threat of the IRA, it didn't stop us enjoying ourselves. We did have to learn to be observant though, and make sure that no-one left unattended bags or luggage anywhere. It was a habit that most people living in London developed and many people checked under their cars before getting in them as car bombs were a common form of attack.

Brenda was loving being back in London, but she missed her family. They had moved to Ireland, as her dad worked for Waterford Glass in the very south of the country. She was close to her family and talked about them a lot. I had met her mum when she had visited Brenda in Leicester while she was on her adult placement there. She was a larger-than-life woman who insisted on hugging me the first time we met, which was a bit awkward as I didn't come from a demonstrative family.

The weekends with Brenda were fun and we explored London together, visiting the Natural History Museum and the Victoria and Albert Museum. I liked museums but there had only been two in Leicester, which I had visited ad infinitum. The Jury Wall Museum was my favourite because it had the remnants of Roman walls and baths in the grounds. The contents inside were interesting too but I had seen them so many times, they had lost their interest. The museum was on the way into town from where I lived as a child and I spent many summer days walking around and checking out the exhibits. I think I also went for something to do and somewhere warm to go when it was raining; plus it was free entertainment and I never had any money. Leicester was a big city and did have quite a few activities, but there was no comparison to London.

Brenda was also lucky in that she lived near to central London and everything was within a reasonable distance, which made visiting her all the more exciting.

# Chapter 7

# Consumption

Tuberculosis had once been called consumption, and the term can be found in novels by Charles Dickens. Charles Dickens himself had praised the work of the London Chest Hospital for providing care for people of the East End of London.

People with tuberculosis were nursed in bays in the early 1980s. Prior to that there had been male and female wards for them, and balconies where they could be nursed in the fresh air. There were no longer the large numbers of patients with tuberculosis needing inpatient treatment that there had been in the past. Many patients with the condition were seen in the outpatients' department by Dr Caplin or one of his team. I was told that the tubercle bacillus, (the bacteria called mycobacterium tuberculosis the main culprit responsible for tuberculosis), rose into the air for 48 hours before falling to the ground, hence the high ceilings in most tuberculosis hospitals and the need for fresh air. Interestingly, although I don't think this was known at the time of the construction of the hospital, there were vents near to the ceilings that extracted air, which may have been an unwitting bonus to the design of the building.

The land next to Victoria Park in Bethnal Green had been acquired due to its large plot, and balconies were added onto the wards in the early 1900s to enable patients with TB to recuperate in the fresh air. Tuberculosis had been decreasing in the three decades prior to my working at the hospital, mainly due to antibiotic treatment, and that is why the hospital had moved on to treat other respiratory conditions and heart conditions in the 1960s. By the time I worked there in 1980 it had become part of a special health authority called the National Chest & Heart Hospitals, which also included the Brompton and Frimley Hospitals.

The main problem with tuberculosis, I discovered, was getting the patients to adhere to the treatment regime, which involved taking three different antibiotics for six to nine months. Many patients stopped taking their treatment and began to develop antibiotic-resistant strains of the disease. In fact it was in the 1980s that TB began to rise again due to drug-resistant strains, just when people were beginning to talk of the disease being eradicated. Health professionals may have taken their eye off the ball due to the emergence of HIV and AIDS in the early 1980s.

TB was mainly found among the homeless and the Asian population at that time. The condition had long been associated with poverty and overcrowding, hence its ability to thrive in Victorian Britain and why it was common in the East End of London. It would spread rapidly due to people coughing and sneezing. Interestingly, there were widespread public health campaigns in the early 1900s encouraging people to cough into handkerchiefs, similar to recent public health campaigns to stop the spread of influenza. Unfortunately, they did not have disposable tissues to throw away back then, so it may not have been as effective, but it had to be better than coughing into the air. Hand-washing facilities in Victorian Britain were pretty scarce too. Symptoms included bloody sputum, cough, night sweats and weight loss. Patients would often appear at the hospital looking like they had come straight out of a concentration camp.

When patients presented with classic signs of TB, they were admitted to the ward for sputum samples and chest X-rays for diagnosis, but as it took weeks for the laboratory to grow the bacillus they began the treatment regime before confirmation of the diagnosis. This was the ideal time for us to try to explain the importance of sticking to the treatment, and to explain the dangers of stopping before the treatment had cured them. One of the doctors had given us our TB lectures and instilled into us the importance of spending a lot of time with patients explaining the treatment. The treatment regimes had dramatically decreased in length of time. Treatment had been for two years in the early days of using antibiotics. This was then reduced to eighteen months, then to nine months and finally to six months. This was as a result of developments in medicine and new antibiotics, but it was still a long time for many people (particularly the homeless) to stick to taking multiple medications. The beauty of working in London, and at a specialist hospital, was that we were at the forefront of medical advances and would become familiar with new treatments before they were rolled out across the country.

Many patients were still taking a treatment termed 'triple' therapy, which was given for eighteen-months, but the new treatment regime included just two drugs (although this later became three again, but different drugs). The early triple therapy included streptomycin, isoniazid and ethambutol. Ethambutol had replaced a powder called para-aminosalicylic acid, or PAS for short, and shortened the course of treatment from two years to eighteen months.

The new triple therapy treatment regime that I would become familiar with included isoniazid, rifampicin and pyrazinamide (PZA), and this soon shortened the length of treatment again to nine months and then six months. Prior to the discovery of penicillin about half of people with TB died of the disease.

Brian had been admitted after being found in Victoria Park barely able to stand. His cough was typical of the disease, as was the sputum he coughed up. He was as skinny as a rake; I could count his ribs without touching him, and he looked much older than his thirty-seven years. Sputum samples had been sent away and his chest X-ray showed a consolidation of his lungs that was typical of tuberculosis.

'Right, Nurse,' Dr Mackintosh had looked at me. 'Let's get the treatment started. Can you explain to Mr Durham what is going on.'

It was a statement, rather than a request.

'Yes, Doctor. Come with me, Mr Durham.'

'Call me Brian,' he said. We walked over to the treatment room where I was going to give him his first dose of the drugs and explain the six-month course of antibiotic treatment.

'Right Brian, you will need to take three tablets a day, as TB is treated with what is called triple therapy, which means three different antibiotics. This has been found to be the best way to cure the disease, but only if you complete the course. One antibiotic on its own does not work as the bugs get used to it and start to fight it.'

I showed him the tablets, explaining that these treatments would need to be taken every day in the morning. 'The most important thing you will need to remember, Brian, is that even when you start to feel better, the disease will not have gone, and if you stop taking the medication before the end of the course the TB will come back. Not only will it come back, but these tablets may no longer work or be able to kill the bacteria. Do you understand?' I asked.

'I think so,' he replied, 'but that's a long time. I'm very forgetful, particularly when I've had a drink.' I knew he had been found in Victoria Park and that he was homeless. Many homeless people did have drink problems.

'Brian, you are still very young, and TB is a horrible disease which can make you feel terrible, as you have already discovered. People die of it.' I waited for this to sink in. 'So you are going to need to remember, no matter what else happens. Dr Macintosh has arranged for you to go to a hostel for a while after you leave here and they will help you to get into a routine as well.'

'Yeah, maybe, but I prefer to look after myself.' I knew what that meant; he preferred to drink himself into a stupor. He was already suffering some tremors and they were not just as a result of the TB infection.

'Give the hostel a chance; you might even like it,' I smiled. 'Anyway, you don't need to think about that now because you will be staying with us for a while yet, while we get the treatment started.'

Many young men like Brian had left home and moved to London thinking that the streets were paved with gold, only to find that they brought their own problems with them. Whatever they were running away from, they were unlikely to find a haven in London's East End, where they were targets for criminals, or where they couldn't find work and ended up on the streets. Try as I might, I got the feeling that Brian was unlikely to stick to the treatment regime; but I was going to give it my best shot, just in case.

Funnily enough, although I came across many patients suffering from tuberculosis in the two years that I worked at the London Chest Hospital, I never came across one as bad as the young man who had died in Leicester. Special had been absolutely right when she said I would never see a chest X-ray like the one I had seen back in 1979.

Special and I wrote to each other for about five years after I left Groby Road Hospital in Leicester. Her letters were short and to the point, letting me know what was happening on the ward and how the staff were doing. They were never personal, but I got the feeling I had become family to her. I am not sure whether she had any other family, and she didn't socialise at the hospital. This was not surprising as she scared most people to death. I'm not quite sure when we stopped writing, I guess time just took over and life became so busy. It is one of my regrets that we lost touch. I think I last heard from her when she was retiring, and perhaps without the ward stories to recount there was nothing much else to say. She did enjoy hearing my ward stories for a while and she shared her love of gardening, something a young girl in her twenties was unlikely to enthuse about.

Bart, the physiotherapist, was always around on the chest wards, mainly carrying out chest physiotherapy, although he did do some mobility exercises too. His main task in life though was to help patients to clear the gunge from their chests, and as I said before, this was not something he could do alone, so we were all trained in how to carry out chest physiotherapy. Bart was a lovely man, always cheerful; we would hear his cheery voice as he came onto the ward and he brightened up our day. The patients loved him, except when he was battering their chests, that is. He would tell them funny stories in his Chinese accent and make them laugh.

One day, a crowd of us were in the canteen when Bart came in. 'Hi girls,' he called, frowning slightly as he saw Martin sitting in the corner reading his Bible. He came and joined us for lunch. 'How's it going?' he asked.

'I'm knackered,' said Jen. 'I can't sleep, there's always too much noise. I'm not used to it. In Stornoway all you hear is the birds in the morning. Here it's loud voices, banging and clattering of doors, and loud music.' At this point she glared over at a girl on another table who was obviously the music culprit. Before she started to wax lyrical about the beauties of Stornoway again, May piped in.

'I am loving the cardiac ward; it's so interesting. I'm sick of hospital food though.'

'I have an idea,' Bart replied. 'Why don't you come over to our flat next week for dinner? My partner's a chef.' Excitedly, we all accepted the invitation and agreed the following Wednesday when we were all on earlies. Bart gave us the address.

The following Wednesday we all pitched up at Bart's flat and the door was opened by a man about twice the size of Bart, with curly brown hair.

'Hi, I'm Charlie.' We had thought Charlie was a girl, and it took us a minute or two to allow this to sink in. Bart was obviously gay, although the term wasn't used back then; we would have said homosexual. I have to say that Bart was the first openly gay man I had ever met (relatively open at least), and they made a lovely couple. Charlie was indeed a chef, and we were treated to the best meal we had eaten since arriving in London. A month or so later, Bart looked very glum when I saw him on the ward.

'Are you okay?' I asked. He had tears in his eyes.

'Why don't you and the others come over for dinner later this week and I'll tell you.'

Jen, Fran, May and I managed to agree an evening when we were all off and we went to Bart's. Charlie answered the door again but he too looked glum.

'Oh dear, they must be splitting up,' whispered Jen.

We ate another wonderful meal and then Bart broke the news, holding Charlie's hand as he did so.

'My father is ill; he is dying.' We all made sympathetic remarks. 'As I am the oldest son, it is my responsibility to provide for the family. Its tradition,' he smiled weakly. 'There are no government benefits in China and my family will have no money if I don't return. I have given in my notice and I leave for China in three weeks.' We all stared, aghast, hardly knowing what to say. Being totally unfamiliar with this type of culture there was nothing we could say. One thing we realised immediately, though, was that Charlie would not be going with him.

'I couldn't live in China,' Charlie explained, 'and even if I could, Bart's family would never accept me; or us as a couple.' We got that; it was hard enough in this country, but in many parts of the world it was much worse for homosexual men. All we could do was express our sympathy, and it was genuinely meant. We had become so fond of Bart; he was part of the furniture at the London Chest Hospital and his happy demeanour and friendship would be a great loss.

On the way home we discussed the evening's turn of events. 'That's really sad,' said May. Even though her vicar's daughter upbringing couldn't quite allow her to embrace the homosexual thing, she genuinely liked the couple.

'What an awful thing to happen. I didn't realise other countries didn't have a benefits system,' responded Jen. We looked at her with incredulity and wondered where she had been all her life – *Stornoway*, of course.

'I will miss Bart,' chimed in Fran. 'He really helps me with the chest physio and he's a great teacher.'

'What an incredibly unselfish thing to do,' I said. I couldn't imagine being that dutiful myself.

Bart did leave, returning to his own country never to be heard from again, and I don't know what happened to Charlie. We went to his leaving do, which was held at their flat, and although we had plenty to drink it was a fairly sombre evening. We went home feeling like we had been to a funeral, and I guess, in the grand scheme of things, it was pretty much like that.

Another patient I had met who was suffering from tuberculosis was Mrs Flavin. Mrs Flavin had been sent to us from casualty at the London Hospital not far away after suffering from worsening breathlessness. Her chest X-ray showed pleural effusion, and because she had tuberculosis the hospital was concerned that the effusion would contain tuberculosis. They were correct in this assumption as it had indeed contained the bacillus.

A pleural effusion is where fluid enters into the lining of the lungs, and it can be small or large; occasionally it can occur around both lungs if congestive cardiac failure is the cause. In Mrs Flavin's case it was around the left lower lung lobe, and because it was causing severe breathlessness, the consultant had ordered a chest drain to be inserted. We had been taught about the procedure in lectures and I had experienced measuring contents of numerous chest drains, but had not seen one inserted. Staff Nurse Blenkinsopp had suggested I assist for the experience. *Why do they feel it's necessary for students to see everything?* I muttered to myself unreasonably.

Dutifully, I had set up the trolley, and I knew I wasn't going to like it – never mind that Mrs Flavin would probably like it even less.

'At least she would be less breathless at the end of it; what is in it for me?' I mumbled.

'Experience.' Staff Nurse Blenkinsopp had crept up behind me and heard my mutterings. Sometimes I really did think I was too squeamish for nursing, but I always came back for more. Doctor Reynolds was the registrar who worked on Dr Caplin's team at the time, and he was a born and bred Londoner.

'Right, Nurse, let's get on with it.' *If you insist*, I thought, but turned to Mrs Flavin.

'Right Mrs Flavin, we just need to turn you over onto your right side so that the doctor can put the drain in. It shouldn't take too long and you'll feel much better afterwards.'

I had already closed the curtains around the bed and I then helped her into position. It was a sterile procedure so Dr Reynolds was gloved up, but because TB was also involved we were both gloved, gowned and masked once Mrs Flavin was in position. Dr Reynolds painted the whole of her left side with iodine before doing anything. I passed him the syringe, needle and local anaesthetic solution, and he injected an area between the ribs. Then came the gory bit. I opened a long plastic tube which contained a thick metal spike, like a knitting needle but much sharper and much thicker.

'Ok, Nurse, support the patient,' instructed Dr Reynolds, and I went around the other side of the bed to support Mrs Makin, holding her hand to reassure her and myself. I was glad she was holding my hand. Thankfully Dr Reynolds was really good at the procedure; I observed quite a few junior doctors later who were not nearly as adept. It takes quite a bit of force to get the spike through the chest wall, between the ribs and into the pleural cavity. Once he was certain he was in the correct place, he pulled the contraption out, leaving the tubing in place with a clamp over it. The tube was then attached to a pressurised bottle about the size of a large plant pot with water in the bottom, and the clamp was removed. Before long, pus, blood and gore were draining into the bottle, and Mrs Makin was starting to breathe a bit more easily.

'Thank you, Doctor,' the sweating patient and nurse said in unison, me thankful it was over and Mrs Makin thankful she could breathe again. Antibiotics were started and Mrs Makin was sent for a chest X-ray to make sure the tube was definitely in the right place. The chest drain bottles were measured daily until it was time for their removal. Occasionally one had to be changed if it became full or lost its suction.

Mrs Makin made a good recovery, and continued treatment for the tuberculosis until the disease was cured. I know she was cured because I met her again in outpatients a few months later, and we reminisced about the chest drain episode. Surprisingly, she said she hadn't noticed that I had been squeamish at all – another case for RADA then. For those who don't know, RADA is the Royal Academy of Dramatic Art in London, where budding actors and actresses go to study. Every nurse could also be an actress.

'I thought you had seen it performed a thousand times before, Nurse,' she said. 'I just hope I wasn't squeezing your hand too hard.' *Or I, you,* I thought. 'It'll be nice not to be treated as an outcast anymore.' Mrs Makin remarked, and I realised that patients with TB suffered more than just the physical symptoms of the disease; there was still a lot of fear surrounding the condition.

Infectious diseases do tend to frighten people into somewhat irrational behaviour at times. TB was one of many conditions that people were worried about catching – not surprising when considering its history.

# Chapter 8

# Making Ends Meet

I soon realised that either living in London was costing far too much money or I was spending too much. Whatever the cause I was not just broke, I was way more overdrawn than usual. So much so that I received a letter from the bank manager enquiring about my overdraft – in other words telling me to sort my finances out. Receiving a letter from a bank manager at twenty-one is a scary experience, and one that was not to be ignored.

He was absolutely right; I had been going out far too often and living on fast food which should have been free, considering the health problems I was likely to incur in later life, but unfortunately it wasn't. The proximity to the West End of London and all its attractions was too much for me, and that, coupled with going out with the girls to the Bonner a few times a week, had taken its toll on my finances. In addition to this, Brenda lived close to central London and she had much more money than me, and always wanted to go somewhere to eat or to a show. The list of shows I saw in London is way too long to go into but I saw Evita in its early days; Educating Rita; Jesus Christ Superstar and many more besides.

The theatre was a lot cheaper than it is now, but it was still pretty expensive, costing about a quarter of my weekly salary. Then there were the art galleries and museums and *Madame Tussauds*. I was never going to have any money. Thankfully I discovered classical concerts and the opera later, otherwise I would have been in even more debt. Brenda's favourite eating house was the *Hard Rock Cafe* near to Marble Arch. I loved it too, being an Elvis fan, but it wasn't cheap.

The bank manager's letter brought me down to earth – I was not a tourist on permanent holiday, I was a nurse earning a very low income. I also felt bad that I hadn't been home at all since moving to London, but there was no money for train fares on top of my living the high life. No, it had to come to a halt. No more jaunting off into the West End every time I had a day off. I still wanted to go out to the Empire in Leicester Square a couple of times a month though, and Thursday night at the Bierkeller near to Trafalgar Square was definitely not going. The Bierkeller was the highlight of my Thursday evenings when not working – we all sat on benches at really long tables in the cellar of the building. There we drank German lager by the jug-full and joined everyone waving glasses in the air while singing songs all evening at the tops of our voices. They don't do nights out like that anymore.

I decided to join a nursing agency and work my days off and some evenings. I found an agency called London & Provincial Nursing Services and they had offices on Regent Street, so I applied to them for work. They snapped me up, and soon I was being booked in for shifts all over the place. The pay was better than what I got for working at the hospital, as higher hourly pay was the perk that attracted nurses to agency work. My first few shifts were at St. Thomas' hospital.

St. Thomas' or Tommy's as it was known, was set back next to the River Thames, across from the Houses of Parliament. It has been a London landmark for years due to its proximity to Parliament. I was very excited at being able to say I'd worked at Tommy's, which was seen as being really posh, and Tommy's nurses' were well thought of in the profession. The reality though, was that it was just like any other hospital, with scary ward sisters and sick patients. The main difference was that the nurses thought they were a cut above the rest and the patients could be a bit more demanding. I had been booked for a late and an early shift on a surgical ward where they were short staffed. The nurses and many of the patients spoke with posh southern accents. The majority of patients I'd met so far at the London Chest Hospital had cockney or Asian accents.

I felt a bit like a fish out of water as I didn't know anyone, and because I was an agency nurse they were not going to spend time getting to know me; I was there to do all the jobs they didn't want to do. At least it wasn't for the most part emptying bedpans though, because they needed me to do dressings rounds and 'obs' rounds. I found it difficult at first not knowing where anything was, and when I did find the equipment room I had to make multiple trips, because the dressing packs didn't contain everything I was used to. It was also difficult because I didn't know who any of the patients were. I had been given a list of people I needed to see, but it was not in any sort of order. The ward staff were obviously busy and short staffed, hence my presence, and sighed every time I asked them anything. I also stood out to both patients and staff because my uniform was different. I wore the London & Provincial uniform, which made me stick out like a sore thumb.

I was getting to the point where I thought I would never finish anything, when a student nurse came along.

'I've finished my jobs; do you want me to help?' I could have kissed her.

'Yes please; I don't know who is who.' Bryony turned out to be a great help and a good laugh too. She had a good rapport with the patients as well, and made them laugh with her Irish brogue. Bryony attached herself to me for the rest of the shift, which is not surprising as the staff nurse who was on duty was obviously too posh to wash, or do anything else for that matter. She sauntered up and down the ward examining her nails as if admiring a freshly performed manicure, and sighed every time anyone spoke to her.

'That's Snail,' explained Bryony. 'She is always on when it's busy and because she is so slow, it gets ten times busier, as everyone else has to do double the work.' As if to reinforce what Bryony had just told me, Snail slowly turned around and walked back down the ward again, having achieved absolutely nothing.

'Hello Mr Bronson,' Bryony turned to the next patient on our list. 'We are just going to take your stitches out.' We closed the curtains and Mr

Bronson entertained us with tales of his family life. It was lovely being back on a surgical ward where people came in, had surgery, and for the most part got better and went home. I realised that I had only been on medical wards so far at the London Chest Hospital. I was yet to move to the cardiac and chest surgery wards. Mr Bronson was an absolute gentleman and couldn't thank us enough as we left to go and change the trolley for the next dressing.

'You've got some nice patients on this ward,' I remarked. In fact, in my experience the majority of patients did their best to be pleasant. There was always the exception to the rule, and for some you couldn't do anything right, but they were not common.

'We have,' Bryony agreed. 'I have met a few awkward ones and some very demanding ones, but for the most part I am enjoying it. The staff can be trying though; Snail is a pain but Sister Proud who you will meet tomorrow is a nightmare. We call her Jaws.' *Oh lovely, just when I thought I had left that type of sister behind in Leicester.* Bryony and I went to break together and she told me how she had moved from a big Irish family farm in Ireland to London.

'At first, I was scared,' she said. 'I wasn't sure how people would be with us Irish, what with the troubles and all, but the girls in my set are lovely. That's perhaps not surprising because we have girls from all over the world, including Australia and Singapore.'

'My set are all from the UK now although some weren't originally,' I said, 'but we do have staff members from all over the world. London is so cosmopolitan isn't it?'

'I had never seen a coloured person until I came over here,' Bryony said. The term "coloured" was not an offensive term in the 1980s, and was in general use as a polite way to refer to people who were black and to people who were Asian.

'Really? I grew up in Leicester, and we have areas that are predominantly populated by Asians and parts that are predominantly populated by Afro-Caribbean people. There's a fantastic area for buying Asian food too. It's not without its tensions though; in fact in Leicester, when I was growing up, there were frequently fights on a Saturday night between black and whites, whites and Asians and black and Asian. I have never understood why people fight over the colour of their skin.'

'We have the Catholic and Protestant thing,' said Bryony, 'and that probably beats the lot.' With that, we decided to talk about nicer things and compare notes of places we had been to in London. Bryony was only eighteen, and had not been to as many places as I had, but she had perhaps explored more of the cultural elements of London. She told me about the Houses of Parliament and the changing of the guard, and I realised, much to my surprise, that I hadn't been to see Buckingham Palace yet. I resolved to do so at the next opportunity, because at least it was free to go and watch the changing of the guard and stand outside the Palace gates. Apart from being an attractive building, I wasn't very interested in going inside the Houses of Parliament though.

It was difficult getting into central London the next day to start the early shift at Tommy's, and I had to wake at the crack of dawn. I then found myself standing sandwiched on a tube train for the whole journey with hardly an inch of space between myself and the next person. So this was the London rush hour that everyone spoke of – I couldn't believe how ignorant people were. No-one stood for elderly people, and men sat on seats while women stood. This was unheard of in my world. Every time the train stopped at a station, more people crammed in. I didn't think it was possible for anyone else to get onto the train, but on they came, elbows first, and somehow they managed. I was fascinated by this early morning activity and looked around, surveying the scene. It was as if everything was happening in a dream. Nobody spoke, nobody looked at each other. Men read newspapers, balancing on briefcases while holding onto an overhead rail, or standing sardined into position by those around them. Women read books or magazines and some carried Walkmans with music tapes inside, with earphones on their heads. Prior to the invention of Walkmans it was not uncommon to see people carrying around

Ghetto Blasters, much to the annoyance of the many.

The majority of people on the tube were wearing suits of some description. I had my uniform in a rucksack and was wearing jeans and a bomber jacket, not that anyone noticed. I suddenly realised that I could die on that train and nobody would notice or even care. For the first time since moving to London, I had found something I didn't like. For a moment I imagined my respiratory patients trying to breathe in an environment like this and realised it would be impossible – as it was I was having to breathe shallower than normal due to the close proximity of a rather large man.

I was very much relieved to finally arrive at Westminster tube station and get off the train, except that everyone else got off too and I was carried along with the throng. I wasn't sure I was heading in the right direction, but I realised that even if I had wanted to go another way, it would not be possible. People weren't just walking, either; they were marching, verging on a trot. Hundreds of faceless people marching to who knows where. I was carried along to the escalator and crammed onto that too. Many people were trying to walk up the right-hand side as it was traditional on the Underground to stand to the left if you wanted to be carried up the escalator, allowing room for people to walk up or down on the right. This could be quite amusing at times when people who didn't know this rule, usually tourists, were thrust out of the way by some impatient Londoner. There wasn't a lot of walking going on that morning, due to the delays at the top of the escalator caused by people trying to exit using the ticket barriers.

Once at the top I managed to grab hold of a wall and stand for a minute to get my bearings. I realised I was going where everyone else was so there was nothing for it but to follow – or be dragged along with the crowd. "Follow the crowd" took on a whole new meaning to me that day.

The day didn't get any better, as Jaws was eating student nurses for breakfast; even Bryony made herself scarce. I was told to go and help with the breakfasts, do an 'obs' round and then change the intravenous infusions (IVs) that were due. Snail was on duty as well but didn't seem to go any faster with Jaws on duty than she had the previous day, although she wasn't quite as visible. I was still recovering from the tube journey and so no task could faze me today. I was dreading a repeat of the morning, realising that I would be finishing shift at rush hour, so was delighted when Bryony suggested going to a pub across the river after work.

After that first initiation to the London Underground in rush hour, I did get used to the crush, as I worked many agency shifts in central London. It wasn't long before I too learned to stand on a tube train without holding onto anything and read a book on my way to work for those shifts. *If you can't beat them, join them.* I did always stand for elderly people though, as that was something I couldn't get out of my system. My mum had taught me as a child to always stand for adults (women at least) and the elderly. Some habits, I believed, were worth cherishing, and that was one of them.

I worked agency shifts at a number of London Hospitals, including The Cromwell Hospital in Kensington, which was a brand new private hospital, opened in 1981 where I was later offered a job. The rich and famous were treated at the Cromwell, many of them from overseas, and its state of the art facilities made it a dream to work at. It remains private but has changed hands a few times. The footballer George Best died at the Cromwell long after I had stopped doing any shifts there.

I also worked in some patients' own private residences. I worked regularly at a lady's home in Kensington; she was a frail old woman who didn't really need a nurse, but she felt she did. On the first day I arrived at a large Victorian terrace with the customary multiple steps leading to the door. Think *Upstairs, Downstairs* and you will get the picture. The door was answered by a cook, who showed me upstairs to a large drawing room where a tiny, grey-haired and immaculately dressed lady sat on an enormous settee.

'Hello, Nurse, I am Mrs Bellings. There is a list of jobs for you over there; it is cook's day off and I don't like to be alone,' she continued.

I checked the list and couldn't believe my eyes – I was here for eight hours and all I had to do was check her blood-pressure, pulse and blood sugar (she was a diabetic) and provide her with tea at 11am, lunch at 1pm and tea at 3pm. *Doddle*, I thought. I almost felt guilty about being paid for the privilege. Mrs Bellings looked at me. 'I don't want you hanging around up here with me. There is a sitting room for you downstairs.' *Even better*, I thought. Mrs Bellings turned out to be a delightful 80-year-old aristocrat (she was titled) with a razor sharp mind. I think, had Agatha Christie met Mrs Bellings, she would have based *Miss Marple* around her. Her diabetes was well controlled with twice-daily insulin and a carefully crafted diet made by cook. She did like the odd biscuit or two, but I didn't dissuade her from this, her only vice. Her husband had worked in the City of London, that small area where the whole country's financial markets are traded. He had died five years prior to my meeting her and she missed him dreadfully. She wasn't a demanding patient at all; in fact, I used to sometimes try to get her to be demanding.

Mrs Bellings liked tea made in a pot with one ordinary teabag and one Earl Grey mixed in, and she would only drink from china cups with saucers and spoon. I developed a liking for the tea mix and occasionally, when I use a teapot these days, rather than a bag in a mug, I make this mix and smile with fond memories of Mrs Bellings. The other treat she was partial to was a giant mushroom, with butter, baked in the oven.

I worked regularly at Mrs Belling's home throughout my training for three reasons. Firstly, the work was light; secondly, I was able to study around her minimal routine; and thirdly, I liked her. It worked well for both of us. Sometimes cook would change her day off around my shifts because she knew the old lady liked me.

Thanks to my agency nursing shifts, the bank manager was happier – at least I think he was (he never said) but he stopped writing to me, and I was able to continue to enjoy the treats that

London had to offer, albeit in a slightly trimmed fashion.

# Chapter 9

# Chugging Along

The most common form of cancer that I came across at the London Chest Hospital was lung cancer. Mr Robinson had given us our lung cancer lectures over a few weeks.

'Now ladies, I am going to teach you the symptoms of lung cancer in a way that hopefully you will remember.' He then bent over with his arms by his side, and gradually started moving his arms round and round in a rhythmic fashion, pretending to be a train.

Jen nudged me and whispered, 'He's flipped; can happen to anyone, you know.'

I was beginning to agree with her when he started to make chugging noises like a train starting up, which then got faster and faster. After a short while he replaced the chugging noises with a rhythmic recitation of, *'Cough, sputum, dyspnoea, pain, haemoptysis; cough, sputum, dyspnoea, pain, haemoptysis; cough, sputum, dyspnoea, pain, haemoptysis,'* interspersed with, *'loss of weight is often late.'*

I can still see him now standing at the front of the class. Soon we all joined in, and he was right: I have never forgotten that lesson and I doubt any of us ever did. He taught us this in roughly the order that the symptoms develop in lung cancer, with the cough often being the earliest symptom.

Lung cancer was often diagnosed too late, meaning that the prognosis was poor. Treatment was limited back then anyway, although some patients did survive. Each type of lung cancer was determined by its cell type, and all but one was associated with smoking. I remember looking long and hard at my cigarette during break after this lecture, and I tried giving up about three times while working at the London Chest Hospital. The first time I tried to give up was after meeting Brian.

Brian was admitted to the ward for bronchoscopy. Bronchoscopy involved introducing a flexible tube with a light and camera attached to it into the lungs. The doctor, usually a consultant at the time, could then see any suspicious areas in the lung and take a biopsy. This biopsy was sent away for histology testing to look for cancer cells. We were one of the major centres for lung cancer treatment in the East End of London and therefore it was not uncommon to see a disproportionate number of people with the disease. This tended to skew our view a bit, and it was difficult sometimes not to imagine that everyone had lung cancer, which of course they didn't.

Brian was forty-three years old with a wife and two young children, aged ten and seven. He worked in a brewery in south London. He had been a smoker since he was fourteen, and had developed what he called a smoker's cough about a year prior to admission. Six months later he noticed he was coughing up sputum, and more recently he realised he was becoming breathless. He had shrugged it off, telling his wife that he was out of condition, but she insisted he go to the doctor when he started to cough up rusty sputum in the mornings. His chest X-ray had shown a small shadow in his right lung and he was admitted for tests and bronchoscopy. His results came back showing he had oat cell (small cell) carcinoma (cancer) which was one of the worst and most common forms of lung cancer.

Cancer was rarely spoken of with patients initially and it was usually a relative that was told first, but Brian had asked the consultant, Dr Bright, to be honest with him, whatever the results. I was with Dr Bright when he came to see Brian and his wife, Grace, on the ward. Children were not allowed to visit the ward because the risks of them picking up infection were too great. Brian could see by Dr Bright's face that it was not good news.

'I'm sorry Mr Blake, I have bad news for you.'

Dr Bright was better than most doctors I had come across in these situations, who would usually blurt out in clipped tones, 'It's cancer you've got,' or: 'Hard luck, it's cancer,' but Dr

Bright allowed his first bit of news to sink in before proceeding.

'You have lung cancer.' Another pause while he allowed the news to sink in. Grace was welling up by this time and there was a deathly silence. I could hear myself breathing.

'Unfortunately, it is not one we can operate on, but we can offer you cytotoxic drugs.' Cancer chemotherapy was in its infancy and sometimes experimental at this time. Patients were rarely given a choice about treatments back then either. They were told what was available and it was generally assumed that they would go along with it, even though they did have to sign consent forms. 'We can start treatment tomorrow. I will see you then.' Dr Bright sighed, shook Brian's hand and then left.

Brian was silent. I could tell he was processing the information and could see the fear in his eyes, but he was trying to comfort Grace. 'Don't worry, I'm in good hands aren't I, Nurse?' He looked at me.

'The best,' I said weakly, remembering the prognosis that Mr Robinson had taught us in class. Months, not years, he had said. Patients rarely asked about prognosis in 1980 as things were just not discussed openly. It was a time when everything was bottled up. It made it a lot easier for us healthcare professionals in many ways but on the other hand it was really difficult. We knew, and usually patients knew, that their end was near, but we didn't talk about it. Some relatives would ask the doctors in private and some would not. Nurses didn't usually give out the bad news in those days either; it was almost always doctors, and most of the time they were not very good at it.

After Grace left the ward that afternoon I noticed that Brian was just staring into space, unable to comprehend that a week ago he was at work and now he was facing his mortality. It was impossible to imagine how he was feeling, but anyone with a bit of empathy could have a good guess. Fear, anger, regret, family, children, why me? I went over and asked him if I could get him anything.

'I need a cigarette. Is it worth stopping now?' he asked. Smoking was not allowed on the wards at the London Chest Hospital but there was a designated smoking area for patients. Thankfully, it was a rhetorical question as I would have wanted to say *no it's not* at that point, but couldn't have said it out loud.

'I think I'll just go for a walk if that's okay?'

'Of course,' I said. 'Do you want company or would you rather be alone?'

'Company please,' he said and after letting the ward sister know where I was going, I followed him off the ward. We got downstairs to the ground floor and went outside onto the front lawn where there were benches. Brian had on his slippers and dressing gown and I was in my short-sleeved uniform. Thankfully it was a warm rather than cold spring day, a bit chilly, but nothing I couldn't manage. We sat on a bench and he got out a cigarette, and just held it in his mouth without lighting it. We sat in silence for a while and then I asked him how he had met his wife.

'I was doing a delivery at a pub in Hackney and I saw this beauty come out with a couple of other girls. She took my breath away and I nearly dropped a barrel on my foot. I was in her way and so she had to look at me. I was just turned thirty and recently split up with my fiancée; she was twenty-five at the time. I smiled at her and said, "Do you come here often?" It was the only line I could think of, and I was dazed. She laughed and said that was original, and before I knew it we were chatting over a barrel of beer. By the end of the conversation I had asked her out and we arranged to meet at that pub the next night. I was smitten. Do you believe in love at first sight?'

*No I did not. Lust at first sight maybe, but not love*; however I replied, 'I'm sure it happens.'

'It does and it did. From that night on I knew we were made for each other; I had never felt like that with my fiancée. We had drifted along together and started living together without ever discussing it. In fact we never discussed anything, and finally we drifted apart in exactly the same way, without any discussion. With Grace though it was entirely different. I knew I wanted to spend the rest of my life with her.' Realising what he had just said, he welled up and then he looked at me. 'I just thought it would be a lot longer.' I put my arms around him and he cried and cried and cried. I thought he would never stop, but finally he did and then he sat up.

'Sorry,' he said.

'You have nothing to be sorry for,' I managed to say, as I was beginning to well up now. It started to rain, and we looked at each other – twenty-one year old me and this man whose world had just come crashing down.

'Come on,' I said, 'better get inside.' I stopped myself saying 'before you catch your death'.

It was one of those moments that I look back on and think what a privilege it has been to stand by people at the most vulnerable times in their lives. Even when it is impossible to cure or heal them, the next best thing is to be able provide a strong shoulder to cry on. After that conversation with Brian, I remembered back to my interview at the start of my nursing career and how I had no idea why I wanted to nurse, but when asked the question I had replied that I wanted to provide support people when they were ill, when they were vulnerable. That answer, though contrived at the time, was inspired, because it became the backbone of the reason why I continued to nurse. As was often the case, the strong shoulder wasn't that strong, and when I went off shift that afternoon, I cried alone in my room. I decided to give up smoking immediately, after I had finished the next packet, of course.

Cancer chemotherapy was fairly new to the hospital and was given in clinical rooms. The senior sister, who was one of the God squad, administered chemotherapy and often spoke to people about God. Some of the staff thought this was dreadful, touting religion when people were vulnerable. One such person was Steve.

Steve was doing agency shifts at the hospital when I met him. He was quite short at five foot six inches, had wavy, long blond hair and lovely blue eyes. He was also an Enrolled Nurse; he had moved up to London from the south of England and was doing agency shifts to supplement his income while working at King's College Hospital full time.

We met when I was working on Hilton Ward, which was the second respiratory ward in the hospital. We hit it off straight away and it wasn't long before we were sort of dating. I say sort of because I was already going out with someone else, a Turkish chap called Mustafa who was probably way too old for me anyway, and I was also trying to avoid an amorous taxi driver who had decided I was the one for him after dropping me off after a night out. Mustafa and I had met in a pub across the river; as soon as my friends and I walked in, he made a beeline for me. By the end of the evening he was asking if he could see me again and we drifted into a fairly platonic (on my part) relationship. On the Sunday before I met Steve, Mustafa had taken me to Petticoat Lane market – an incredible place which was absolutely jam packed. It was also a haven for crime, so I had to keep my handbag close at all times.

Petticoat Lane is a famous market in the East End of London, popular with tourists, and I believe that Alan Sugar started out there as a stall holder. Stalls sold just about everything you could think of, including a lot of stolen goods, and it made Leicester market seem small. The unusual thing back in 1980 was that it opened on a Sunday, as most markets were closed on Sundays.

Mustafa had insisted we have our photo taken with a little monkey on my shoulder. The monkey was similar to the one in the film *Raiders of the Lost Ark*, which I saw a few years later. I was starting to tire of Mustafa as he was a bit too clingy for me, and although I don't think he had marriage in mind given that his family would want him to marry a Muslim, he certainly had other things in mind. It had been a convenience relationship and I had decided on that Sunday that I would not be available in the future.

There was a marvellous night receptionist/porter called John who used to keep my admirers at bay, as sometimes I found it difficult to turn down dates. John would ask me who I was happy to see and then tell anyone else I was working or out, and he would also shield me from telephone calls. John and my friends used to laugh at the predicaments I got myself into, and there were some tricky moments when more than one guy would turn up at reception at the same time. I am ever grateful to John, who became a good friend and who taught me that it was ok to say NO. Men would get over it, he told me. John, himself was engaged to a lovely girl called Laura and I had met her at their engagement party in the spring.

Steve and I seemed to be getting along really well, and he was certainly the most interesting man I had met since moving to London, although he was a bit moody. He could be really interesting and we would have deep conversations, but he could also be quite negative. He basically had a chip on his shoulder and felt that he was owed a living because life had given him a hard time. From what I could tell, the only hard time he had was that he had to work. His parents were well off, but his father had made it clear to him that he should make his own way in life before being given any handouts – he resented his father for this and so had become a nurse because he thought his father would disapprove. In actual fact, his father thought it was a good thing to do and that he would learn some discipline. Needless to say, once Steve got onto this subject he became very pouty. I can't say I had a lot of sympathy as my upbringing had been far harder than his (not that we were comparing), and I never felt that the world owed me a living. It's odd how different people can be, but I still liked Steve very much until one day when I was going back on shift after a lunch break, and met him on the stairs.

'THAT WOMAN,' he shouted, 'is preaching to people who are terminally ill; she should be sacked.'

I knew straight away he must be talking about Sister Blair, the senior sister from one of the wards who administered cancer chemotherapy. I was a bit tired.

'So what?'

'It shouldn't be allowed; these people are weak and vulnerable and she's taking advantage.'

I could see his point in one respect but then again, I could see hers; what if she was right? 'I'm sure they can make up their own minds,' I said, starting to get slightly irritated with him. I was more irritated with him shouting at me about something that had nothing to do with me, even though I knew it was because he was frustrated and he couldn't shout at her. On top of that he was a confirmed atheist, and had really taken a dislike to the God squad from the word go. He was one of those people who hated anything to do with religion, not in a normal way but in a very aggressive and unreasonable way.

'They shouldn't have to listen to that crap when they are dying,' he continued in a very loud voice that was starting to draw attention to us; and now people thought we were having a row.

'I don't see how telling people that God loves them when they are dying can be so wrong,' I replied. 'Anyway, can we talk about this later, I need to get back to work.'

'Arrogant cow,' I heard him mutter loudly as he walked off, and I hoped he wasn't referring to me.

That was the last I saw of Steve; he never did any more shifts at the London Chest Hospital. I was a bit sad because I liked him but boy was he volatile. I have no idea why I defended Sister Blair, who I didn't even like that much as she was a bit too much like Martin, a bit too intense for me. Having seen many people near to death who would ask about life after death, and actually wanted to talk about spiritual things to which I never had the right answer, I thought that maybe she was just fulfilling a need rather than imposing her views. Steve was overreacting to hearsay, I thought, although I would never know, and nurses could indeed be sacked now for proselytising to patients. I couldn't understand why Steve was so angry, but for some people, religion is an absolute taboo subject whereas others will gladly discuss the matter. I wondered if I had reacted differently, whether Steve and I would have developed a deeper relationship, but then if he could fly off the handle over something I was not responsible for; what would he be like if it were something I had done?

I am not sure what Sister Blair said to patients but none of them ever complained about her to me. Some would laugh and call her the nun and others would actually want to know more and request a visit from a clergyman. We did have people of other religions in the hospital, in particular Muslims and Hindus, but I don't think she overtly tried to convert them.

When administering cytotoxic drugs, Sister Blair would wear theatre-type clothing and a big rubber apron, a bit like those worn by pathologists. She would also wear double gloves, a face mask, a hat and goggles. This was all to protect herself from exposure to these very toxic drugs. She was quite small, like me, and the gear she had to wear used to drown her. It was a wonder that this diminutive woman could talk about anything under all of the coverings she had to wear.

In some cases cancer chemotherapy was given as well as radiotherapy and/or surgery. Chemotherapy could be given before or after either of those treatments, but not at the same time. Although I was not able to administer the chemotherapy I did have to care for the patients on the wards, and so needed to understand the treatment and the side effects.

A group of us had got together over a meal with Mrs Chang at Chloe's flat one night. Chloe had invited us all but only seven of us could make it, and as Mrs Chang was coming we asked if it could include some revision – we were all feeling like our heads might explode with all the information we were trying to take in. In addition to this we still had to do our shifts and ward work – not to mention my agency work and night life. A few of the others were doing some extra shifts at the hospital on their days off to earn extra money. I was trying to avoid this as I didn't feel I had enough experience yet; some of the others had worked on intensive care before starting at LCH, so they could do shifts in the cardiac ICU.

Mrs Chang always managed to cheer us up no matter how tired we were feeling, and Chloe's cooking helped – not to mention the wine. Once we had washed up and drunk enough wine Mrs Chang explained to us the importance of observations after chemotherapy. Jen had wanted to know why people lost their hair and May had questioned whether the treatment was any good at all, while I wanted to know why a patient had to wait weeks before being given a second lot. Surely it was better to blast the cancer. Mrs Chang was patient with us.

'The reason for any of the side effects, including hair falling out, is that the treatment hits good cells as well as bad. Tumour cells divide more rapidly than normal cells so it does attack them mostly, but there are cells in the body, such as hair cells and those helping to fight infection, that are affected because they also divide rapidly. That is why there is a decreased resistance to infection and why people's hair falling out is a common side effect. As treatments get better and more research is carried out I'm sure they will become more cancer-specific, but for now we have what we have.'

'That brings me on to my point,' said May. 'What is the point of having a treatment that nearly kills people? Wouldn't it be better to leave well alone?' I did think that May had a point; I had seen well looking patients come onto the ward for treatment. A few days later they were vomiting everywhere, had terrible diarrhoea, developed infections as their white cell count was lowered, and some bled from any orifice, not to mention the hair falling out.

'While we have a treatment, albeit still fairly rudimentary, and it offers hope, we cannot deny people the option. For some it will cure them and for others it will prolong their life,' replied Mrs Chang. She sighed. 'It is better to have a little hope than none at all, and treatments are improving all the time. New drugs are being developed and one day there will be a cure, of this I am sure.'

Mrs Chang was ever the optimist and ahead of her time in many ways. There are cures for many cancers now, and new advances in the treatments over the years have most certainly improved people's chances.

'Some people,' continued Mrs Chang, 'may well decide that enough is enough; and I know that for lung cancer things aren't great at present, although they are improving, but it is up to the patient, not us. If we have a treatment we offer it, explaining the risks and benefits, and then it is up to them whether they decide to take the risk.'

'I still think sometimes the doctors are just experimenting,' May retorted. 'What's the point of an extra few months?'

'It might be during those extra few months that a cure is discovered,' said Mrs Chang. *Now that was a good point.* 'Or it may just give people time to sort family matters out: attend a wedding; see a birthday. Also, some people will always live longer than we think they will and many have surprised us all.' She was right there – I had recently met a seventy-year-old patient called Mr Young who had been told ten years ago that he had six months to live.

'I wasn't going to let that whipper-snapper of a doctor tell me when I was going to die,' Mr Young had confided. 'What made him think because he had been to medical school that he could determine when someone would move off this mortal coil? No, Nurse. Your time's up when your time's up, and that's what I told him.' Mr Young certainly did seem to be a medical miracle. He was riddled with cancer but he just kept on going. A positive mental attitude certainly did seem to help people to live longer. I have met people who should have lived for years, who died within a short space of time after being given a cancer diagnosis, and people like Mr Young who lived far longer than anyone ever thought they would.

My thoughts were interrupted and I rejoined the conversation just as Chloe was putting the kettle on. 'So why can't we mega-blast the cancer then?' I asked.

'Well, that is what happens, mainly because although the patient has intermittent treatment, the doses of the drugs are high. They tried it with a single drug to see if there would be fewer side effects, and there were, but the cancer cells developed a resistance to the drug. The best treatment at the present is to give a high-dose combination of drugs intermittently, because resistance takes a long time to develop, and side effects are less because the bone marrow is given time to recover before the next treatment.' We all looked suitably impressed, even more convinced than ever that Mrs Chang went to sleep reading textbooks.

'Does your husband work away a lot?' Fran asked, putting into words what we all thought. Mrs Chang laughed good-humouredly but didn't answer the question. We loved our little Malaysian tutor; she was so bubbly and so unlike most of the horrible ward sisters from our student days. Mrs Chang never frowned, although her energy was exhausting sometimes. Perhaps it was as well for her husband if she did go to bed with a textbook, as who could keep up with her?

We ended the evening with coffee and cake and were all very happy. Chloe's flat wasn't far from the hospital and it was easy enough for us to walk back to the nurses' home afterwards. Mrs Chang's husband came to collect her in his car and we all tried to see what this man looked like. He appeared Chinese was all we could see in the dark, as he drove away with our lively teacher.

When we got back to the hospital, I joined John behind reception for one of our late night photography chatting sessions. We were both keen photographers, although he was much better at it than me, but we would discuss all sorts of things that would help us to improve our skills. He always had the latest photography magazines too, and we would discuss the latest techniques. I had a Chinon single lens reflex (SLR) camera, which was a Dixons Stores own make, and I had been planning to take some black and white photos around the rougher parts of the East End on my next day off. John gave me plenty of advice about how to get the best shots. Before I knew it we were talking into the early hours, which often happened when John and I got to speaking about photography. I finally decided it was time to call it a day, or should I say a night, and headed back to my room in the nurses' home. As I lay on my bed that night, I thought how great it was to live in London and work at the LCH, in spite of the poky little room, the scaffolding outside and the cockroaches.

Mr Robinson's train demonstration popped into my mind, and I smiled as I drifted off to sleep that night.

# Chapter 10

# Cabbages

As well as its respiratory specialism, the hospital was renowned for coronary artery bypass surgery. Because we rotated around the hospital we all worked a stint on the surgical ward, which was mainly for people recovering from open heart surgery. Jen and May had really enjoyed their stint on the ward and now it was my turn. I would be joined by Fran and Flora for this placement. We hadn't yet worked on the intensive care unit where people went immediately following the surgery, but we had each done a shift in theatre to witness it. This was mandatory for all of us so there was no way out. Amazingly, I hadn't wanted to miss out on this one because it would be so interesting, and not many nurses would ever have the experience.

My turn came one Tuesday morning, and I had been warned by my colleagues that I could be standing for 4-6 hours depending on how the surgery went. Thankfully, Fran and I went in together, and we were not expected to do anything apart from stay out of the way and keep quiet, while observing. The surgeons were used to trainees being in theatre and they did not pay us any attention. There were two surgeons, one to remove veins from one of the patient's legs and one to perform the heart surgery. There was also a registrar who assisted the heart surgeon and a junior doctor to assist with anything else and to learn. There were two scrub nurses and two huge surgical trolleys, one for each of the surgeons. The bypass equipment was quite bulky too, and took up space on one side of the theatre bed. In addition to all of these people there were two anaesthetists, one to ensure the patient was anaesthetised throughout and one to keep a check on the bypass equipment. Then there were a few nurses who were there to provide any additional equipment that the doctors or scrub nurses may need. The theatre was pretty packed and there was not much room for Fran and I to position ourselves so that we could watch the procedure.

'Ooh, isn't this exciting?' whispered Fran.

'It would be more exciting if I could see,' I replied. Fran had the advantage of an extra seven inches on me as she was five foot eight whereas I was five foot one. The patient had been brought in by the anaesthetist and everyone had gathered around the bed in their green theatre gowns, masks, gloves etc. It wasn't long before the patient was covered in green sterile sheets and I couldn't see a thing through the sea of green. I spotted a stool on the other side of the theatre and decided to go for it while everyone was busy setting up.

'I'm going to get that stool,' I whispered to Fran, and I started to slowly move around the edge of the theatre, making sure I didn't touch anyone who was wearing a sterile gown. The stool was almost in my grasp when one of the theatre nurses went for it at the same time as me – our heads cracked and we both yelled. Everyone turned to see what the noise was.

'Ssshhh,' hissed the theatre sister.

It was hard to tell who was who as you could only see eyes, but then I noticed that the heart surgeon's eyes wrinkled in laughter. He then put out his left hand and said, 'scalpel,' and carried on. With attention moving back to the real action, I whispered an apology to the theatre nurse and made my way back, minus the stool, to Fran, who was laughing behind her mask. I was rubbing my head and noticed the theatre nurse doing the same.

'That hurt,' I muttered.

'Never mind,' said Fran, who was now watching the surgery. The stool was still in place over the other side, as neither I nor the theatre nurse had picked it up. I decided against a second attempt, particularly as the surgeon was now opening up the chest – or I assumed he was because I couldn't see. I was getting bored because I was just standing there and all I could see was the sea of green theatre cloth. I couldn't even watch the surgeon removing the vein from the leg, as he was on the opposite side to me.

'What's happening?' I whispered to Fran.

'Mr Brown is just about to open up the sternum.'

I saw him pick up a saw, and as the noise of it started to ring through the theatre I took my chance. In a move that James Bond would have been proud of, I was round the other side of the theatre, returning with stool in hand without anyone noticing. With my prized possession in hand the sawing stopped; I was now as tall as Fran and could see what was happening. I saw the surgeon insert the cannulas that were attached to the bypass machine. Blood was then transported via various tubes, filters and a gas exchanger for the next hour, leaving the heart almost empty of blood, allowing the surgeon to perform the bypass. The heart was stopped by reducing its temperature.

I was fascinated as I watched the skill of the surgeon; as he cut the vein that had been removed from the leg into three, he stretched each one out and inspected them like choosing a prime steak. Once he had chosen the best bits he applied the grafts to the affected blood vessels supplying the heart. When the surgery was complete, the heart was restarted and the bypass machine removed. In this instance the patient's heart went back into a normal rhythm straight away.

I hadn't realised while the procedure was taking place how much tension there was in the room, as everyone was on high alert in case anything went wrong. Once the bypass was discontinued, the surgeons, sister and anaesthetist started to chat about golf and Wimbledon, which had just started. It was the summer of 1981.

'Do you think McEnroe will beat Borg this year?' asked the anaesthetist, while the surgeons were busily pulling the patient's sternum back together. McEnroe had lost to Borg in the final the previous year.

'No, I think Borg will win.'

'You cannot be serious,' replied the anaesthetist, mimicking McEnroe's pouty expression and swan song of the time. Everyone in the theatre laughed, and conversation continued in this vein until the surgery was finished. The patient was then transferred to

Intensive Care, where he would be ventilated for twenty-four hours or so following surgery. The surgery had taken six hours, and as I stepped down from the stool, I realised how tense the muscles in my legs, neck and shoulders had been from concentrating.

'I'm starving,' Fran complained.

'Come on, let's go and get something to eat.'

Our shift was effectively finished, as we had been in theatre for an hour before surgery and an hour after helping with the clear up. We hadn't had a drink or anything to eat since we started at eight o'clock that morning. We made our way to the canteen as there was nearly always food there. There were some leftovers from lunches but very little choice, so we opted for sausages and chips.

'That was fascinating, wasn't it,' Fran remarked.

'It was once I could see.' We both laughed, remembering the head clashing incident. 'I've got a lump on my head, feel here.' Fran felt my forehead.

'You have as well, lucky you didn't get a black eye.' We both laughed again. Caffeine and food were starting to revive our energies after what had been a long day in theatre.

'I couldn't do that every day.'

'Me neither; you'd end up with varicose veins, standing in one place all the time.'

'I would never remember what instrument to give him. Did you notice how he just held his hand out sometimes and sister placed the right instrument in his hand without him even asking?' I said.

'I guess she's seen so many of the same operations, she could probably do one in an emergency,' remarked Fran.

'I'm going to Wimbledon on Saturday.' I changed the subject.

'Really? I don't really like tennis to be honest. Who are you going with?'

'Cally.' I replied, and Fran frowned. Cally was one of the God squad.

'You be careful.'

'It's not an infectious disease,' I laughed. 'We haven't got tickets, but Cally says if you go early enough and queue you can get ground tickets.'

That is what happened, and I remember having a great day out on a lovely, sunny June day in 1981. We queued for around three hours, had our bags searched and then saw Stan Smith play in the doubles and also John McEnroe. Stan Smith did get through to the doubles final that year but lost to McEnroe and his partner. McEnroe also beat Borg in the singles final. Cally was nice; she was definitely a born-again Christian but not as intense about it as the others in the hospital. We had sensible discussions as I was interested in the whole thing. I was impressed by the way she lived her life, but felt deep down she needed to get out more. Time would tell whether I was right.

I made two new friends while working on Lister ward. Holly was from Buckinghamshire, an overweight, lively girl with long, dark hair. She was doing the SRN/RN version of the training which was identical to ours. Holly spoke with a posh accent, as did Tina. Tina was also doing the SRN version of the training and originated from the north of England. I got on really well with Holly and Tina but they didn't really get on with each other, so I had to go out with them separately when we socialised.

Tina had a car, which was a rarity in London, so we could go out a bit further afield in the East End. We often went to a pub across the river from where I lived in the nurses' home. Tina lived in a flat not too far away. One night Tina dropped me off back at the hospital, and I was just getting out of the car when Mrs Lumumba came flying out of the front entrance of the hospital, almost falling down the steps.

She started waving her arms in the air like Shirley Bassey, but the arm-waving lacked the Shirley aplomb.

'Nurse Bates,' she shouted. 'I'm your nursing officer – TAKE ME HOME!' With that, she flew down the steps and got into Tina's car. Tina looked horrified. I was laughing my head off, without letting Mrs Lumumba see me, of course. Tina scowled at me and drove off. She later related that it had taken a while for Mrs

Lumumba to remember her address, and even when she did, she didn't know the directions. Poor Tina – she was totally unimpressed at being commanded by a drunken nursing officer to provide a taxi service. I remembered the conversation with Jen of a few months before, and had to admit that Mrs Lumumba certainly liked a drink. She did have her uniform on but I had no idea whether she was on duty or not, and I didn't ask. I think she may have had a drink problem, but it was more than likely confined to the end of her shifts, as there was never a smell of alcohol when she came onto the wards, and she always behaved appropriately.

Tina was not happy when I saw her the next day, fuming at the audacity of the woman she had been made to drive around London for ages, looking for an address in an area that she didn't know. I didn't say much because I was secretly fond of Mrs Lumumba for giving me the opportunity to move to London, and found the whole thing amusing – but then I was not the one who had been accosted in the hospital forecourt so I could afford to laugh.

Many patients who came to the London Chest Hospital for heart surgery were local NHS patients, but quite a few came from abroad, paying privately for surgery. Wealthy Indian and Pakistani men were treated and operated on. It wasn't just foreigners who paid privately; we also had wealthy businessmen from the UK who were treated privately. This was not unusual in the NHS, where consultants would undertake private work in addition to their NHS duties. I'm not quite sure where all the money went other than in consultants' pockets, as none of it came into the hands of other NHS staff, who provided the majority of the care. One such wealthy businessman was being cared for on Lister and I was checking his 'obs'.

'Do you like cocktails?' he asked.

'I like most drinks,' I replied. He reached over into his bedside locker.

'Here,' he said, and handed me a ticket. 'I was given a ticket to a business cocktail-tasting party taking place in Bow, but as you can see I won't be able to attend,' he smiled.

'Ok, thanks,' I said, and put it in my pocket. It could hardly be considered a bribe, since it was a free cocktail party. I looked at the ticket when I got off the late shift that night, and realised it was for the next day, at 5 o'clock in the afternoon. Formal wear, it said on the ticket, and business people only. I wasn't going to be put off going to a cocktail-tasting party on a minor technicality, and I decided to go. Sadly, it was for one person only so I couldn't take any of my friends. The next day I put on my interview clothes, as these were the only decent clothes I had. A beige, brown-speckled skirt and a light brown blouse. It was a warm day so I didn't need a jacket, and I walked along to the venue with the aid of a map and a few stops to ask directions.

I arrived at a small hotel and entered confidently, seeing the sign for the cocktail-tasting event in the foyer. I followed the sign and handed my ticket to the person on the desk. Fortunately, there were lots of people entering at the same time so they didn't really look at me, otherwise they would have noticed that I was the youngest person in the room.

The room was lined with tables in a U shape and a rectangle of tables in the centre, meaning that there were tables to the left and the right as I started along the route. The cocktails were laid out in cocktail glasses, about a third full, which was perhaps as well. I was doing nicely, and was on my fourth taster when a man in a business suit sidled up beside me.

'What business are you in?' He looked at me sceptically. I put on my posh voice and replied that I was in computers – hoping that he knew nothing about computers because I certainly didn't. We still hand-wrote everything, including our case studies, and the only computers I knew were cardiac monitors and the like. I continued along my way, trying to ignore him, but he was determined.

'What type of computers?' he asked. 'You look very young.'

'Yes, people who develop computers are very young. It's my father's business.' I was astonished at how easily I was able to fabricate stories. I think that one I did inherit from my dad. 'To be honest, I like to forget about them when I'm out. What business are you in?' I tried a different tack. It worked because he was now in his element.

'I'm a banker.' Yawn, yawn, I was still off bankers with the letter from my bank manager fresh in my mind. He started talking about investments, stocks and financial markets. I think he might have even given me a few share tips, but I wasn't listening. I was flying around the room drinking cocktails, while he was following me, continuing in full flow. *Was he never going to tire of his own voice?* Twenty cocktails later (I think), I thought it was time to leave and said goodbye to my banker shadow, who was still singing the praises of financial markets. *Really, he needed the cocktails more than me.*

'Nice to meet you,' he finally said. 'Whoever you are.' I knew he hadn't believed my story and I can't say that was surprising as I had always looked even younger than my now twenty-two years, but I didn't really care. At least I was out of the door and I had enjoyed my outing. It would have been a bit nicer if I could have taken more notice of what I was drinking, but it had been a pleasant experience. I'm not quite sure how I managed to walk back to the nurses' home that night, but I had certainly had an interesting diversion. I made a mental note for the future to always have a story at the ready, and eat before ever attending such an event again. Alas, no-one has ever provided a free cocktail-tasting ticket since.

Mr Williams was admitted to Lister ward for cardiac catheterisation with a view to surgery. He had been suffering from angina as a result of coronary artery disease for four years. His angina had worsened and he was also very breathless. When I first met him, he was really overweight for his relatively short stature of five foot six inches. He seemed much older than his sixty-six years.

I could tell he was really anxious on admission, and his mobility was poor; he was brought to the ward in a wheelchair.

'Hello Mr Williams, I am Nurse Brookes,' I introduced myself. 'That is Mr Fogherty in the bed next to yours, and on the other side is Mr Jones; across the other side of the bay are Mr

Black and Mr Fox.' All of the patients smiled at him apart from Mr Black, who was not a friendly man.

'Don't worry,' said Mr Fogherty in his thick Irish accent. 'The nurses are nice and the food's not half bad.' He winked at me. Mr Williams attempted a smile. His wife had accompanied him to the ward.

'I'll close the curtains and leave you to get into your pyjamas.'

'Thank you, Nurse,' his wife smiled; she had told me that she would stay with him for a while and help him get settled in, because he was such an anxious man. She was used to doing most things for him at home, including wheeling him around in a chair they had purchased. After he had changed into his pyjamas I returned, armed with the nursing care notes that I needed to complete in order to admit him to the ward. He was quite breathless, though some of this was due to his anxiety and once he felt more at ease the breathlessness improved. I wrote in his notes that he would need reassurance. I was looking at his medical notes while I admitted him, and one of the doctors had written that he was a 'whiner'.

The days of doctors writing rude remarks in patients' medical records was almost at an end, but not quite. Medical notes were confidential, and some doctors felt it gave them the right to say what they liked about patients. It wasn't unusual to see patients referred to as 'fat' or worse – ignorant; paranoid (when they were just worried); time-wasters and all sorts of other things. Sometimes they could be regionally insulting, using the letters N.F. in front of the initial letter of a town or area – translated as 'Normal for...'. Not all doctors did this, and hospital doctors were often the mild offenders compared to GPs who could be downright rude – even in their admission letters, which would sour the minds of ward staff towards a person. Sometimes what they wrote had truth in it, and sometimes it was just their interpretation. Doctors' letters to each other both from and to the hospital could begin with words such as:

'This very nice young woman'

'This neurotic woman'

'This obnoxious man'

'This fat, lazy man'

'This charming gentleman' and so on. These judgemental remarks said more about the doctor than they did about the patient, because the vast majority of doctors rarely strayed away from the polite and professional, keeping their letters and records objective. Nurses, too, could and would write derogatory remarks in their records, but this was less common, as most ward sisters and matrons would come down on them like a ton of bricks.

I checked Mr Williams' observations and they were normal, apart from a faster than usual respiratory rate. I realised that he would not be able to breathe with the standard two pillows, and went to fetch him three more so that he could be well propped up when in bed. I asked Mr Williams about his medical history.

'Mainly this angina, Nurse; I did have an appendix out when I were a youngster,' he informed me. 'The only other time I was in hospital was when I broke my ankle playing football in my twenties.' It was hard to imagine

Mr Williams ever being my age, but of course he would have been. I often found it sobering when meeting patients to imagine that they, like me, were once youngsters, and that they all had lives outside of the hospital wards. I found it did me, and them, good to ask about their lives in most cases.

'What did you do for a living?'

'I were a plasterer until five years ago. I had to give up when this angina started up.'

'Are you from around here?' I continued.

'I was born in Southend and have lived there all my life except during the war. I'm a home-loving man really; met the wife at a party when I were twenty-three. It took me most of the night to pluck up courage to ask her to dance, and then I trod on her toes for the rest of the night.' Mrs Williams obviously didn't mind as she agreed to marry him when he proposed. 'We were married in June 1938,' he said proudly. 'The next year we declared war on Germany and I was drafted for military service.' Most men between the ages of eighteen and forty-one were drafted.

'Where did you go?' I asked. The men in the surrounding beds were all sitting up listening now as they were all war veterans too, apart from Mr Black, who had a heart murmur and had been refused entry, which hadn't helped his attitude any.

'I was signed on for the navy and worked in the engine rooms of a submarine; I was also taught to fire torpedoes.'

'I was RAF, flew spitfires,' chipped in Mr Fox.

'Were you really? I was RAF, air traffic control.' Mr Jones joined in the conversation. Before long, they were all reminiscing about their wartime escapades and reminding themselves how lucky they were to have returned intact. Mr Fogherty had been in the army and had been stationed in Singapore for a while.

Mr Williams had returned from the war to be reunited with his wife, and they had two boys who were now both married with children of their own. He was delighted to have two grandsons and a granddaughter, and he had spoilt them rotten prior to his condition worsening. He said he found it difficult now because they wore him out, but he still loved seeing them.

The next morning Mr Williams was taken to the cardiac catheterisation lab for coronary angiography. This procedure involved inserting catheters into a vein and an artery, then a dye was inserted and the coronary arteries were filmed on a screen by a specialised camera. The outcome for Mr Williams was that he had severe blockages to his coronary arteries. He was seen by the consultant, who explained the problem and offered him surgery. Mr Williams agreed to the operation, and returned home with an appointment for surgery in the following February. He seemed much happier on discharge.

'I feel like something can be done now,' he explained. 'Before it was like being in a dark tunnel with no end in sight, whereas now I have hope. The doctor said that my symptoms will be a lot better after surgery and that I could live a normal life.' His eyes lit up as he told me this and I realised again how easy it was to judge people when they were vulnerable. Many patients with chronic illnesses suffer depression and anxiety as a result of their symptoms and the debilitation they cause, and while some are able to remain positive, not everyone can. It was lovely seeing him so happy, and he even said he was going to try to lose some weight before surgery as the doctor had advised him to. He had already given up smoking just before admission, and this would help his symptoms too.

On the same day that Mr Williams had gone for his angiogram, Mr Fogherty had gone to theatre for coronary artery bypass grafts – known as CABG and pronounced cabbage. I had found it really confusing when I first started working at the hospital and people kept talking about patients and cabbages.

'We had three cabbages today,' remarked Fran.

'That's a lot of cabbages – why?' I had asked. Fran had looked at me a bit strangely. 'Because they needed surgery.'

'What has surgery got to do with cabbages?' Suddenly Fran, Jen and Blanche realised we were on different wavelengths and they burst out laughing.

'Cabbage, coronary artery bypass grafts, Dawn – CABG,' laughed Jen.

*How was I supposed to know? Silly hospital acronyms.* I had joined in the laughter once I got the joke. Everything is easy when you know. It wouldn't be the first time I mixed up acronyms – it's a bit like singing the wrong song lyrics for years and then realising.

Mr Fogherty lived in London's East End, where he moved for work following the war. He had worked in the building trade for many years until he developed angina in his sixties. In spite of the damage to his coronary arteries he continued to smoke, which was not uncommon, much to the despair of cardiac surgeons. It was at this time that I began to question my own hypocrisy – advising people to stop smoking while I continued to smoke myself never sat comfortably with me. As I said previously, I attempted to stop smoking myself on at least three occasions but didn't manage to last longer than a couple of months.

Mr Fogherty was married to his childhood sweetheart and they had four children, two boys and two girls. One son was a teacher, the other was a plumber, and his daughters were married with children. One daughter was a social worker who had moved to Leeds some ten years previously; the other was a part-time shop assistant and mother who lived in Guildford. The family remained close, and met up at least once a month. There were eight grandchildren. I had got to know Mr Fogherty quite well since he had been admitted for surgery.

Two days prior to surgery, he was visited by the anaesthetist, who examined him and prescribed his pre-medication. On the day of surgery he was given valium 20mg orally at six o'clock in the morning and then intra-muscular omnopon and scopolamine at seven o'clock. He was also given intramuscular antibiotics that would continue for ten days. I had shaved Mr Fogherty's chest and leg the day before and explained to him that he needed a pubic shave. 'I can do that myself, Nurse.'

'You might not be able to see properly but don't worry Mr Fogherty, Nurse Brown will do that for you.' Alan Brown was an Australian male nurse who had recently joined the hospital, working on a twelve month visa. Mr Fogherty looked relieved; it would have been embarrassing for him to have a pubic shave from a snippet of a girl, as he used to call me. Alan also assisted him with the iodine baths that were part of the pre-operative regime for two nights prior to the operation and on the morning of surgery. I had given him two glycerine suppositories the night before surgery to ensure his bowels were empty. So many procedures had become routine to me over the past few years. It was hard to imagine that innocent young eighteen-year-old who had first started nursing four years before and at twenty-two, I had seen and witnessed so many things that most people may not witness in a lifetime. For the most part I counted it a privilege to be a nurse, although sometimes I wished I didn't have to see so much illness, heartache and death.

Thankfully, when one of us was down because of some trauma we had witnessed, the others would help us through it. On that particular morning when Mr Fogherty was in surgery, Mr Fox called me over, saying he felt unwell. He was pale and clammy, and I was about to call the doctor when he collapsed back on the bed.

'ARREST' I shouted, while feeling for a pulse and checking for breath all at the same time, and one of the nurses ran to fetch the resuscitation trolley while I removed the pillows and commenced cardiac massage. I asked one of the patients to pull the curtains.

In every hospital at the time there was a special cardiac arrest telephone number which was dialled, and then all the on-call doctors would get an arrest bleep, which was usually a rapid, continuous bleep. They would get to the nearest telephone to find out where the arrest was and then come running. This whole process happened in minutes, which I was grateful for because cardiac massage drained energy fast and was stressful. Alan was on duty, and he brought in the resuscitation trolley and applied a face mask with a bag attached to it to administer breaths to the patient when cardiac massage paused. After a few minutes the first doctor arrived and then an anaesthetist; they took over the resuscitation and then shouted their instructions. They would shout for various drugs used to assist with restarting the heart and set up the defibrillator. Resuscitation techniques have improved dramatically over recent years, and defibrillation is given much faster as this is usually what saves lives. I had grown attached to Mr Fox, a gentle seventy-year-old man who was due to go for surgery the next day, but at that time I was working on adrenaline. As the team continued to try to bring this man around though, the adrenaline wore off and I realised that they were not going to succeed.

During cardiac resuscitation there is a moment when realisation sets in that it is not going to be successful, and a hush replaces the frantic activity. Usually resuscitation was attempted for at least an hour, but when that moment comes it is horrible. The doctors and nurses exchange glances and then the doctor will usually shake his/her head and all the work will stop. The doctors then look at their watches, agree time of death and walk away back to rounds or clinics. The nurses are left with a chaotic mess and a dead patient. Alan and I looked at each other and then slowly started clearing away the mess. I looked at Mr Fox with tears in my eyes.

'I'm sorry that we couldn't help you, Fred.' It was the first time I had called him by his first name. I held his hand for a moment, which by now had turned cold. Fighting back tears, I helped Alan clear up the resuscitation trolley and tidy up the bed. The nurse in charge had called his family and they were on their way to the hospital, not knowing yet that he had died. Alan and I also had to re-stock and re-check the resuscitation trolley, accounting for all the drugs that had been used so they could be replaced, and double check everything. As we emerged from behind the curtains Mr Black called, 'I've been waiting for my painkillers for an hour,

Nurse, and my bed hasn't been made this morning.'

'Bl...y wait,' Alan muttered under his breath.

'I'll bring them in a minute, Mr Black,' I replied, uttering the same sentiment under my breath. 'Your bed will be made when there is time.'

As soon as we had finished checking the trolley, bells were ringing and the nurse in charge called 'Hurry up, Nurse. The lunchtime medicines need to be given out now. We are running behind.'

'Oh dear,' I turned to Alan. 'How could Mr Fox have been so inconsiderate? Did he not realise there were beds to be made and medicines rounds due?' I chanted sarcastically. Alan smiled grimly. We understood that a death on the ward affected some more than others, and we continued with our jobs.

Mr Fogherty returned to the ward two days after surgery, and he was so relieved to be back his euphoria spread to the other patients. It was the lift we all needed after the death of Mr Fox. Mr Fogherty was a new man; although he had post-operative pain he was ecstatic at being given a new lease of life. Mrs Fogherty was also ecstatic, and this pleased him too.

Post-operative care included four-hourly 'obs', chest physiotherapy three times a day and deep breathing exercises. He also had steam inhalations four times a day. These were given through a white pot called a Nelson's inhaler – named after the doctor who designed it. Boiling water was poured into the container and then a cork stopper put in place. The cork had a hole in it to allow tubing to be placed inside so that the patient could inhale through this. There was a spout to allow the steam to escape and reduce the risk of burns.

A chest X-ray revealed that he had developed collapse in the bases of his lungs following surgery.

'He'll need the Bird, Nurse,' the doctor said to me.

The Bird was a machine that provided assistance to patients to expand their lungs via a process called intermittent positive pressure ventilation. It was quite common for patients to develop lung base collapse, because they found it difficult to breathe deeply due to the pain from surgery. The Bird, if given four times a day, would push a mixture of air and oxygen into the lungs and expand them. I explained the process to Mr Fogherty.

'The physio will show you how to use the machine,' I told him.

'I don't mind, Nurse, I'll do anything to get better,' he smiled.

'That's good,' I said, 'because you will be mobilising from tomorrow. Time to get you moving again,' I laughed. The next morning I helped him walk to the bathroom and got him a chair to sit on at the wash basin.

'It is so long since I've been able to walk very far,' he confided. 'I have been an invalid with the wife doing everything for me.' After his wash I wheeled him in a chair to the dressing room and took off his dressings. Both the leg and the chest wound were healing nicely.

'There's just a small bit of oozing at the bottom of the chest wound,' I told him. 'I'll put a dressing on that but the rest we can leave open now.' I also helped him to put on a white anti-embolism stocking, which took a lot of heaving and pulling on my part. He would need to wear the stocking for three months, I told him.

'Good job my mates won't see it,' he laughed. It was lovely watching Mr Fogherty become a new man every day – he was his old self again, said his wife. The only time he was reluctant to move was around the fifth day after surgery, when all the bruising came out. Once he knew this was normal, though, he soldiered on, and by the end of ten days he was ready for discharge. His lungs were back to normal, his stitches were all out and the antibiotics finished. He opted to go for convalescence, and was discharged to Frimley Park Hospital. I was absolutely ecstatic to see him leave the hospital in a far better state than before. The surgeon had not really considered him a good candidate for the operation but he was as pleased as everyone that it had been a success. Mr Fogherty would no longer be a cardiac cripple, and he left the hospital full of hope.

I had learned more lessons again as a nurse, and gone from an extreme low following the death of Mr Fox to euphoria following the transformation of Mr Fogherty. The highs and lows were something that I never totally got used to; I didn't like the emotional swings, as they didn't suit my personality. Nursing was always going to be emotionally challenging though, but it was at times like this that I knew why I loved the job.

# Chapter 11

# The Smelly Shoes Episode

The second medical ward I worked on later in the year was called Hilton. This is where I got to meet my friend and member of the God squad. Sister Wright was in her late twenties, average height with dark brown hair tied up in a ponytail. Cally was a quiet, almost shy, unassuming woman who went about her work in a professional manner. I didn't get to know her well initially, but by the end of my placement we had become good friends, along with a staff nurse trainee called Lottie, short for Charlotte. Lottie was also a church goer, although she didn't call herself a born-again Christian; she had been brought up in the Church of England and was an Anglican. I was still quite ignorant in my understanding of all of this as I thought in terms of Catholic and Protestant, and was only just discovering that there were all sorts of denominations relating to Christianity. It was all very confusing for an agnostic.

Whilst working on Hilton ward I met Miss Smith, a thirty-eight year old lady who was admitted to the ward for chest investigations. I was the admitting nurse, and on taking her history I discovered that she worked as a private secretary to a bank manager. I was tempted to relate my story of letters from the bank manager, but decided against this. Miss Smith was single, and stated she was happy to be so as she enjoyed work and travelling. She had travelled quite a lot, visiting many countries including the USA, Barbados, Australia, Israel and Mexico. She had two older brothers who were married, and her parents were elderly but well. Miss Smith was a non-smoker and her only problem prior to this admission was that she had suffered from chronic sinusitis since the age of twenty.

Miss Smith said she had suffered from a chronic, dry cough for about ten years. Her GP had told her that this was due to the sinusitis and had advised her to have antrum washouts, which she had refused. Again, I resisted the temptation to relate my recent experience of antrum washouts, and my meeting with Robert the Bruce.

About two weeks prior to admission she had developed a persistent cough with what we in the profession term purulent (lots of) sputum. Her GP referred her to us for investigations. From the outset, Miss Smith made it clear she was not happy about being admitted to hospital, but I think it was more out of fear than for any other reason. After all, she hadn't met Robert the Bruce.

After filling out most of the paperwork, I checked her temperature, pulse, respirations and blood-pressure. We were still using mercury-filled thermometers and sphygmomanometers. A sphygmomanometer, or 'sphyg' as we called them, was used to check blood-pressure. They came encased in a hinged, rectangular wooden box. When the lid was opened you could see the mercury-containing measure attached to the lid. An arm cuff was placed around the upper arm of the patient and then, whilst inflating the rubber cuff by squeezing on a hand-held rubber ball, we had to use the other hand to apply the stethoscope over the brachial artery in the mid-arm. This procedure had taken many attempts to learn when I was first training in Leicester, and we had practised on each other until we got it right. It was the dexterity required that had been difficult to master. The other thing we had to learn was to resist the temptation to over-inflate the arm cuff, as it could be painful and patients would complain. Not that we minded when we practised on each other in the classroom.

Anyway, with the skill long since mastered I discovered that Miss Smith's blood-pressure was normal. Her temperature was raised slightly, so she would have four-hourly TPR taken, but daily BP. Her parents had come down from Manchester and were staying in a London hotel not too far away.

After the doctor had examined her and requested blood tests, he also requested that four sputum samples be taken; three to be checked for infection and one to be checked for cancer cells. I gave her four small, sterile sputum pots and explained that she needed to cough the phlegm (as she called it) from her chest into the pots. Miss Smith was also sent for a chest X-ray. This showed a patchy shadow in the left lower lobe of her lung, and the doctor decided that it was suggestive of bronchiectasis. He then arranged for her to have a bronchograph the next day.

I had never seen a bronchography before, and so was encouraged to go with Miss Smith. *I really thought that it would be alright not to see everything*, but Florence would have turned in her grave at my cowardice, so I tried to sound enthusiastic. I was beginning to think that specialist nursing wasn't for me as I progressed through the course and got more and more involved with specialist treatments and tests.

I was still recovering from assisting Doctor Reynolds with the chest drain episode, even though some time had passed since then.

The doctor had explained to Miss Smith what the procedure would entail, and she had taken it all in her stride, unlike me, who was going to have another sleepless night wondering if I would pass out.

The next morning I did manage to turn up. I had considered throwing a sicky, but Jen had told me not to be such a baby. We were in the Bonner the night before.

'It's a simple, straightforward procedure,' she had said. 'I've watched a few times now – it's nothing that Sweeney Todd couldn't have done.'

*Yes, that was really helpful.*

'Thanks for that Jen. Anyway I've decided to write up Miss Smith for my chest case study if she gives me the go ahead, so that should help me be a bit more objective.'

'That's the spirit,' chipped in May. 'In for a penny, in for a pound; speaking of which, it's your round.' We were in the Bonner, whispering in hushed tones so no-one would hear us. Not that you could hear anything over the juke box and the nattering – you certainly couldn't see very far through the cigarette haze. I slept reasonably well after a few glasses of lager, and woke in the morning with a new determination.

Miss Smith had fasted from midnight, and the night staff had given her the obligatory white theatre gown to put on with nothing underneath. An hour before she was due to go to the X-ray department where the procedure was being carried out, she was given a pre-med of omnopon and scopolamine. The pre-med was given to keep a patient calm before or during a procedure. It's a shame there weren't pre-meds for nurses. I gave Miss Smith a theatre hat to cover her hair, which she duly applied.

I walked alongside the trolley, which the porter pushed into the X-ray department where the bronchograph was going to be performed. Miss Smith had had two days of intensive physiotherapy prior to the procedure, to make sure the lungs were as clear of secretions as possible. Doctor Reynolds was going to be performing the procedure, and he explained again to Miss Smith what this entailed.

'We will put a bit of local anaesthetic into the skin in front of the throat first, and then inject deeper into the throat to numb the area inside. Once that is done we will insert a slightly wider needle so that we can insert a plastic catheter into the airway (trachea).'

*Note that when a doctor or nurse says that something is 'little' or 'slightly wider', always read 'large' and 'much wider'.*

Miss Smith tolerated the procedure well, and actually, apart from the thought of someone injecting anything into my throat, which gave me the heebie-jeebies, so did I. Afterwards the catheter was inserted and an X-ray was carried out to ensure that it was in the right place – good idea. Finally, a contrast medium was passed into the lungs and radiographs were taken while tilting and rolling the patient into various positions. While the catheter was in place it prevented Miss Smith from speaking. She was therefore asked to raise a hand if she was in pain. Once the films were taken, the catheter was removed and a small dressing applied over the area.

The results of the tests did in fact show that Miss Smith had bronchiectasis, where there is an abnormal widening of the bronchi which then becomes a reservoir for secretions and multiple infections. This accumulation causes further widening, and the small sacs in the lungs become baggy and enlarge. The disease in Miss Smith's case was secondary to the chronic sinusitis that she had suffered, but it was confined to the left lower zone, which made her an ideal candidate for surgery.

Dr Reynolds explained the diagnosis, as he was the respiratory consultant.

'You have two options,' he explained.

*That's a rarity*, I thought, *giving the patient options.*

'You can be taught how to perform your own chest physiotherapy and postural drainage. You would need to take a small dose of antibiotic every day to try to prevent infections, and we can treat future infections with antibiotics at a higher dose. The alternative is that you can have the lower lobe of your left lung removed, which is likely to result in a full cure, and you will be able to live a normal life afterwards.' Dr Reynolds and I were shocked that she chose option one, but she obviously had a fear of surgery, as she had previously refused antrum washouts for her sinusitis. Respecting her decision, Dr Reynolds explained that as long as she took the prophylactic antibiotics and carried out the physiotherapy for the rest of her life she could go on living normally.

'Are you sure?' I asked her later.

'Yes, for now. I just can't face the thought of major surgery at my age, but if I can manage the condition myself, I would much rather be in control of my own destiny.' She had a point, and she was an intelligent and determined woman who would likely manage the condition very well. She learned the physiotherapy techniques really well and the physiotherapist was happy that she had mastered them. Miss Smith went home with a very positive attitude and was started on tetracycline 500mg twice daily, which was the prophylactic dose that was effective at the time. Dr Reynolds said he would see her regularly in the first year to ensure that she was coping physically and mentally, and the surgery option was kept open for her if at any time in the future she changed her mind.

Miss Smith had a very supportive family, and she taught me a valuable lesson at the time. For me, the choice would have been to get rid of the disease and take the surgery, but not everyone feels that way and, while there were two choices available, it was right for the consultant to outline them both.

I realised I hadn't been out for a while; work had been piling up and I had been writing the two case studies that were a course requirement. Brenda suggested that we go out to the Empire on Saturday night, and as I was working an early followed by a late, I agreed. We met in Leicester Square and went for a drink first. It was therapeutic to be out dancing again and experiencing some normality, as I sometimes felt I lost perspective when surrounded by sick people all of the time. It was also good to hear about her work at Great Ormond Street children's hospital and the kids she came across. We laughed at the stories of the antics the staff got up to on the ward in order to cheer the children up. There weren't too many antics on the wards at LCH because people were too ill, but we did play tricks on each other at times.

That night, I got a taxi home at around three o'clock in the morning, and after a very quick chat with John I headed back to the nurses' home. I was feeling bright and a bit mischievous. On entering the nurses' home I noticed all the shoes outside of the rooms. We always kept our smelly working shoes outside our rooms in the corridor, because the rooms were small and the stink of sweaty feet was very unpleasant. I had the sudden urge to play a prank and decided to swap all the shoes around, even moving some upstairs. After about an hour, I had moved virtually every pair of shoes on all three floors and, pleased with my work, I went to my room. It was now around five o'clock and I drifted off to sleep immediately.

I was awoken an hour or so later by shouts and exclamations as those getting up for the early shift were stomping up and down looking for their shoes. I could hear raised voices and anger and soon everyone was up, with people frantically trying to find their shoes before going on shift. I was really tired and just wanted to go to sleep, but the racket was too much. Eventually I opened my door, and I could see furious faces all down the corridor. I was feeling a bit guilty now, and also a bit scared that if I owned up I might be lynched. Thankfully I had moved my shoes the night before too, so that I wouldn't be a suspect. *It's always good to have clarity of mind when committing a crime*, I had thought. The only difference was that I knew where mine were.

'Can you believe what some idiot has done?' shouted May.

'What?' I said.

'Some prat has swapped all the shoes around. Of all the selfish, idiotic things to do....' She was marching up and down frantically trying to find hers – she was obviously on an early.

'If I get my hands on the b..... fool that did this – they'll know about it!' shouted Jen from the other end of the corridor.

I could see that some people had found theirs and were heading off to work. 'I think I'll find mine later,' I murmured, and went back to bed. I couldn't help smiling at my handiwork in spite of myself. This was one prank I was never going to own up to though, and I never did. To any former friends and colleagues reading this, I'm sorry; it seemed funny at the time. I did get a little retribution later though as I couldn't get back to sleep and ended up going on shift with a splitting headache – reciprocity.

# Chapter 12

# Flat Time

Brenda had been going on at me for a while to think about a flat share with her and two of her Great Ormond Street buddies. I had met Sharon and Lynne a few times, and we had been out for meals together when I had stayed with Brenda. Sharon was quite posh, the daughter of someone very high up in the Royal Air Force, and Lynne was equally posh and quite unassuming.

I had been living in the nurses' home for almost a year and was soon to be finishing my course, so I needed to move anyway as new students would move into the home I was in. I agreed to join them and we started flat hunting. It wasn't long before we found a first floor flat in a large Victorian semi-detached house in Stoke Newington, north London. The area was populated largely by Jewish people, with the majority of men sporting long beards with long sideburns and wearing black clothing along with rather large black hats. The flat we decided to rent was owned by a Jewish man who lived around the corner.

After living in the nurses' home this flat seemed huge. It had a large kitchen and bathroom, and an enormous lounge. The only downside was that we would need to share bedrooms, but these, too, were huge. We agreed to take on the flat, which was furnished, and would move in a few weeks later. The room that Brenda and I shared was the biggest, and both rooms had twin beds. We all figured that as we worked shifts and were often away (at least, they were often away) that we would manage.

The flat situation worked very well and was quite timely, because we were all qualifying in the near future. Some of my gang were going to be staying on at LCH, although some were moving back home, Flora included. I worked out that I could get a bus from the end of the road to Bethnal Green and so would be able to travel to work by bus and wouldn't need to get a tube. The tube station was a half-hour's walk away, whereas the bus stop was just five minutes down the road. It wouldn't be as easy as walking across a courtyard though.

There were two sisters living in the ground floor flat, and we later discovered that they often had parties, which they invited us to. Sharon spent a lot of time with her fiancé, although there was a little catastrophe when she went on holiday to the Cayman Islands without him and had a fling with a rich man from England who was living on the island. On her return she was convinced she had fallen in love with this man and broke off her engagement, planning to move to the Cayman Islands as soon as she could. Everything about Sharon was very dramatic – she didn't do ordinary at all. Once she got back to work and realised that she really did love her fiancé, the wedding was all back on; Lynne and I took a train to Wallingford in Oxfordshire a year later and witnessed what we had come to term as the Royal wedding. True to form she and her new husband drove away in an open top Bentley.

I had been rather amused when we stopped off at Sharon's home once to find there was a cook and housekeeper, she was obviously used to a more privileged lifestyle than the average nurse.

We spent the winter of 1981-1982 in the flat and one night, after it had snowed, I awoke in the morning to see melted water dripping down the electric light pedestal in the bedroom. Lynne and I were the only ones there so we agreed to go and tell the landlord. It was a Saturday, and the landlord wouldn't answer the door, as they observed the Sabbath to the exclusion of all else. In the end we posted a note through the door, but we didn't see anything of him until the Sunday, and even then nothing was done about the leaking roof for about a month.

One night I was going onto night duty and was waiting at the bus stop when a guy bumped into me. A short time later we got onto the bus, and when I went to take my purse from my pocket I realised it was gone. I walked up to the man, who had also blatantly got on the bus, and asked for my purse back. He just gave me a load of verbal abuse, and I was too scared to do anything more. I felt terrible; I had no bus fare. The bus conductor had seen what had happened and didn't ask me for any fare, which was a great relief. I think that episode put me off living in Stoke Newington. I went onto shift that night feeling quite shaken and violated. I couldn't believe that anyone would steal like that, but obviously people did so. I realised it could have been worse, and that at least I was not harmed. I didn't carry bank cards in my purse to work so he would only have stolen a couple of pounds. It was still my hard-earned money though, and it was not an easy incident to forget.

Lynne met a boyfriend while she was living in the flat, and it became obvious that they were starting to go steady and that she was thinking about moving in with him. Brenda appeared to be going through some sort of personality change, and became moody and a bit hostile, which made her difficult to live with. The forces of nature were at work that would split up our little home after about six months, and everyone would decide to go their separate ways. It was all a bit like the breaking up of the fellowship in the

*Fellowship of the Ring.* Sharon and husband moved to Oxfordshire after she was married and I stayed with them for a short time when I later moved to Reading.

We had some really good times in the flat, and because it was quite large it was great for entertaining; we had lots of dinner parties for friends from both hospitals. Also, it was nice because friends from Leicester could visit, which had been a bit tricky when living in the nurses' home. I think my mum was pleased I was no longer living in the East End of London, although she wouldn't have been so happy if I had shared the bus stop episode.

I had met Robert, a physicist, while working at the London Chest Hospital, a nice man who had not long moved to London himself. He offered to cook dinner for us and came to the flat one evening to make moussaka. I have to say he was a good cook and became a good friend; some time later he joined Brenda and I on a holiday to the former Yugoslavia, where we stayed in a place called Rovinj. We were also joined by a male nurse friend of mine from Leicester, who preferred drinking to tourism. I later introduced Robert to Cally and they ended up getting married.

One night when Cally came round for a meal I shocked her, not to mention myself, when I said I would join her for church one Sunday. I think she nearly fell off her chair, as she had been asking for about six months. I had grown increasingly inquisitive and impressed with the way she conducted herself and lived her life. I was also aware that when being confronted with so much illness and death I frequently felt totally inadequate.

I had recently had a very traumatic experience while working on the high dependency chest unit. This was an eight-bedded unit where patients were looked after following chest surgery. Mrs Frampton was a sixty-year-old lady who had returned from surgery following the removal of a lung. She was doing really well, although still needing a lot of care. Her husband had visited one afternoon and asked how she was, and I had explained how she had coped well with surgery and was stable. He left the hospital at around five o'clock, and one of the doctors came in to change the tubing attached to a central venous pressure line. While he was doing this, Mrs Frampton took a deep breath and collapsed, going into respiratory arrest. We had tried in vain to resuscitate her, but unfortunately did not succeed. I remember vividly her husband being called back into the hospital and, with tears in his eyes, saying to me, 'But you told me she would be alright.'

I felt terrible, not for the first time, and cried myself to sleep that night.

Cally seemed so certain that there was life after death, and she had challenged my lifestyle on a number of occasions. I didn't understand the God thing really, but wanted to see if there was anything to it.

I did go with her to the church she attended in Mile End, and I thought they were all bonkers. There was lots I didn't understand, but I had to admit that they all seemed very happy, and not a drink in sight. As this book is about my nursing career, I will cut a long story short. I was sitting on my rock a few weeks later, and as I looked out upon the water and up at the sky, I felt like I was experiencing the wonder of creation for the first time. I prayed a very raw and amateurish prayer, having never prayed in my life apart from in school assemblies, and I felt different – and, in fact, was different. Obviously my friends had been right to be worried about Christianity being a contagious disease. I won't go into any more detail about this subject here, but I did get a lot of stick from my friends, and my dad was furious. I think he would have reacted better if I had said I had become a prostitute. My mum was alright with it just as long as I hadn't joined a sect that took away all my money. *What money?*

# Chapter 13

# Up, Up and Away

During our final few weeks in training we had taken our last tests and all successfully passed. We had also passed all of our practicals and case studies, so we were feeling very pleased with ourselves. Fran was staying on at LCH to work on the coronary care unit. Jen was staying on for six months to consolidate her learning and then would head back up to Scotland.

We all attended Blanche's wedding in Leicester on the final weekend of the course, and saw that she and Jeremy were absolutely made for each other. It also gave me a chance to see my family, who I had neglected somewhat during my time in London, and to reassure my mum that I was alright. Blanche looked beautiful, and was married in a lively Pentecostal church, showing me once again that the world was raining Christians.

I was offered a job on the cardio-thoracic surgical ward at the Cromwell hospital, which would pay more money because it was a private hospital. I was going to take it, but Miss Bale called me into her office. I had written a letter of notice and thought that she was calling me in to say goodbye.

'Sit down,' she said sharply, and then she scowled at me. I had never seen her angry. 'I could shoot you as soon as look at you,' she continued.

'What have I done?' I asked, astonished by her anger.

She picked up my letter. 'This.' She held it up like a poisoned chalice. 'How could you? We gave you a chance, when no-one else would have. We took you without the qualifications you needed for the course, and this is how you repay us all.' She was quite pink in the face now. 'I will keep this letter for one week young lady.' Miss Bale sat down in her chair looking quite exhausted with all the activity. I realised I was dismissed and left the room.

At first I was angry, but the more I thought about it, the more I realised she was right. They had given me the opportunity, and I had gained all the benefits of the specialist experience. No-one had ever challenged me like this before, but I realised that the least I could do was offer my fully trained skills to the hospital that gave me those skills. I swallowed my pride, said goodbye to the pay rise and backed down, withdrawing my notice. Miss Bale was over the moon, as were Mrs Lumumba, Mr Robinson and Mrs Chang.

'It's not as if you don't like working here is it?' May asked. She had taken a job on the ICU.

'No, I love the hospital, it was only the pay rise and the attraction of living in the West End; but I guess I would have spent too much money anyway.'

We had met up in the Bonner for a last drink before some of the girls left.

'Well I can't wait to get back home,' Flora said. 'Although I will miss you all when I leave here.'

'You won't miss the cockroaches?' Fran teased.

'I do have a bone to pick with you about that,' Flora continued. 'You never did ask anyone to get rid of them, did you?' We all laughed, including Flora.

'Well I won't miss you if I get sick,' Jen said to Flora. The evening continued with good-natured banter. Some of the girls were moving into the qualified staff nurses' home, and others had found flats like me and were living elsewhere.

I ended up taking a job on one of the medical wards, but I did extra shifts around the hospital to keep up my skills. Mr Robinson and Mrs Chang collared me towards the end of the course.

'Dawn,' Mr Robinson smiled. 'Mrs Chang and I both think you should do your SRN training. You will get bored with life as an enrolled nurse, because you are sister material, and that can never happen if you don't do your SRN.'

'Do you think I would get accepted without the educational qualifications?' I asked, remembering Mrs Butcher and my first interview.

'There are a few hospitals that offer the training via entrance exam still,' Mrs Chang replied.

'I have drawn up a list of the hospitals that do.' Mr Robinson handed me a piece of paper. I could have cried. This kindly man and woman both believed in me and were going out of their way to help me. They had no obligation to do this, but I am forever grateful that they did.

I took the piece of paper, and saw that there were about six hospitals offering a two year shortened course for enrolled nurses via entrance exam. They were all out of London, which I wasn't so keen about, but I could always come back, I thought. I applied to three in the south of England, and the first one to respond was Reading in Berkshire. Mr Robinson arranged for me to go and sit the entrance exam at St. George's Hospital in Tooting, as he used to be a tutor there. I did a bit of studying, as I knew from the first time I had sat a similar exam in Leicester that it was IQ-based, with maths and English questions. I was surprised at how nervous I was about it when the day came, but I had now set my heart on doing my SRN training. I needn't have worried; I passed with flying colours. Mr Robinson told me I got 96% and I was thrilled.

I went for my interview at the Royal Berkshire Hospital in January 1982, and was offered a place for the September cohort. I was pleased about this because I could give at least six months work back to LCH after Miss Bale's lecture. Mr Robinson was over the moon, and gave me his old textbooks for when I started. They were too old, but it was a kind gesture from a lovely man.

Tina and I were chatting on the hospital bench in the front gardens of the hospital, as our courses had finished more or less at the same time. I was telling her how pleased I was about getting in to do my SRN (RGN) training, and she suggested a trip to Asia before I started the course saying she had always wanted to travel. It was a timely suggestion, because at that time the government was allowing nurses to cash in their superannuation payments, and I knew that I could pay for such a trip if I did this. We had a short discussion and I agreed. We decided to take a three month trip, leaving in June 1982 and returning at the end of August, as I was due to start training at the beginning of September.

Quite a lot happened in my personal life during the three months prior to the Asia trip. My flatmates were going their separate ways, with Sharon getting married, Lynne moving in with her boyfriend and Brenda deciding she was moving back into the nurses' home. I managed to find a room with a girl from my new-found church, so wasn't homeless. My brother got married at some point and didn't invite me to the wedding, which was disappointing. I think he had forgotten he had a sister due to my rare trips home. On the positive side, I discovered the Royal Albert Hall, the Royal Festival Hall and All Souls Church in the West End. I developed a real love for classical music. I also went to various concerts, and saw Cliff Richard, Chris De Burgh and the Moody Blues.

I continued to enjoy my work at the London Chest Hospital and I was relieved to discover that Miss Bale approved of my leaving to do my RGN training; she even accepted the Asia trip as an acceptable part of growing up. These did not constitute mutiny, whereas leaving her NHS hospital to work in a private hospital did.

Tina and I planned our trip, deciding to start in Singapore, travel up through Malaysia to Thailand and Burma, and then across to Sri Lanka, India, Nepal and Pakistan. Alan had written to an Australian mate in Singapore and arranged for us to go and stay with him and his girlfriend on the first leg of our trip. Tina had told one of her patients about the planned vacation, and as he was from Karachi in Pakistan he offered to put us up when we got there. The rest of the journey we would have to play by ear – staying at guest houses and such like. We found a bucket shop (travel agent) on Regent Street, and went to buy our plane tickets. The only tickets we bought were an outward flight to Singapore, an open ticket to take us from Bangkok to Sri Lanka and a return from Karachi to London, which would be our final destination. The man in the bucket shop gave us the name of his brother, who lived in New Delhi, and suggested we call on him when we got there.

About eight weeks before we were due to fly to Singapore I went to the doctors' for multiple vaccinations. I had been given a typhoid and cholera vaccine, and then gone onto a night shift on the intensive care unit.

Intensive care units are totally different to any other hospital wards because, although there is a patient underneath all of the machinery and tubes, it is the machinery and tubes that are the main focus of attention. The reason for this is that the patient's condition is monitored through the checking of the various contraptions that are inserted and applied. The intensive care unit at the London Chest Hospital had single rooms where patients were ventilated post cardiac surgery. The ventilators in use were pretty basic Brompton-Manley ventilators that had a concertina bellow, which thudded with every breath given to the patient. On this particular night, following my vaccination, I felt myself developing a temperature. My arm swelled up and I was feeling pretty lousy. I could feel myself falling asleep, but thankfully the rhythmic thud, thud of the ventilator and the need to do various checks every fifteen minutes kept me going through the night. There was a cardiac arrest in one of the other rooms that created a commotion in the early hours, and in that case, the resuscitation was successful. Morning came, after what seemed to be an eternal night, and the patient and I had both survived. I was very glad to get to bed that morning after taking a couple of paracetamol tablets.

My final few months of work flew by, and before I knew it, Tina and I were on our way to Heathrow airport, saying goodbye to the London Chest Hospital. I knew that when I returned, another chapter of my life would begin in Reading. I had gone out with those of my friends who still remained before leaving, and had arranged to return to London for a few days after the Asia trip before finding somewhere to live in Berkshire, as there was to be no accommodation for me. Sharon and her husband were living about twelve miles away from Reading in Wallingford, and offered to put me up until I found somewhere closer. That was all I knew as I sat in the Heathrow lounge with Tina, excited about what lay ahead.

We boarded a Pakistani International Airlines jet and were up, up and away.

# Acknowledgements

I have been so encouraged by the comments and reviews from readers of my first book that I decided I had to write the second. I thank all of those people; if it wasn't for them I would have given up on this one many times over. I must also thank the two wonderful tutors that I met during my time working at the London Chest Hospital for believing in me. If it wasn't for them, I would not have pursued the full and varied career that I came to enjoy.

I thank my friends Sue and Ruth for supporting me every step of the way, as always. I apologise for my lack of availability over the past few months and thank you both for your patience.

There are so many people who have inspired and encouraged me over the years, and too many to mention, but here are just a few. Thank you again to Gail for suggesting nursing as a career path. Thank you to my friend who encouraged me to move to London. Thanks to Mr Robinson; your belief in me brought me much happiness, and helped build my confidence in my ability to study. I know there are many others and I thank you all from the bottom of my heart for being friends and colleagues.

As always, thank you to patients, past, present and future; I hope that I have helped some of you. I have learned so much from so many of you; it was always you patients who made it worth getting out of bed in the mornings.

# About The Author

Dawn Brookes initially trained as a nurse in Leicester. Dawn loved her nurse training and wanted to share her memories with others. For some it will bring back memories of either working in hospitals or being a patient or visitor. For others it may offer an insight into what it was like to work in hospitals in the 1970s and early 1980s.

Dawn admits that writing these books has brought back many wonderful memories, and hopes that these come across to the reader.

She moved to London, where this book is based, and then to Reading in Berkshire where she also trained as a midwife. Later, she trained as a district nurse whilst undertaking a Bachelor's degree. She worked as a district nursing sister, then undertook a Masters degree in Education and worked as a lecturer/practitioner. Following this she moved to Derby in order to care for her ill father, and worked as a community matron and, more recently, as an Advanced Nurse Practitioner.

There may be more books to follow in the future. To keep up to date with her work sign up at: http://www.dawnbrookespublishing.com.
See Amazon Author Page to Follow
Contact the author

Dear Reader

Thank you for reading my second memoir, I do hope that you enjoyed reading it. My intention was to provide an insight into specialist nurse training in the very early 1980s and life in London at that time. In order to gain feedback as to whether I have achieved this and any other thoughts you may have; I would love to hear from you either via a review on whatever platform you use or the contact form on my website shown over the page. I am always looking to improve as both an author and a human being and with that in mind I would appreciate your comments.

Yours faithfully

Dawn Brookes

# *Books by Dawn Brookes*

## Memoirs

*Hurry up Nurse: Memoirs of nurse training in the 1970s*
*Hurry up Nurse 2: London calling*

## Nursing

*Non-medical prescribing in healthcare practice: a toolkit for students and practitioners* – Palgrave Macmillan
*How to check blood sugar* (diabetes)

## Property

*Buy to Let: 7 steps to successful investing*
*Property Investment: how to fund your retirement with a buy-to-let property pension*

## Children's Books

*Boats and Ships A to Z: Let's learn together*
<u>Miracles of Jesus Series</u>
*Jesus feeds a big crowd: a very special day*
*Jesus feeds a big crowd colouring book*
*Jesus heals a man on a stretcher*
*Bible stories colouring book 2: Jesus heals a man on a stretcher*

Sign up for newsletter at
www.dawnbrookespublishing.com